HEALTH
CARE
ETHICS

HEALTH
CARE
ETHICS

lessons from intensive care

kath melia

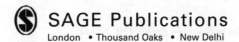

SAGE Publications
London • Thousand Oaks • New Delhi

SAGE Publications Ltd
1 Oliver's Yard
55 City Road
London EC1Y 1SP

SAGE Publications Inc
2455 Teller Road
Thousand Oaks, California 91320

SAGE Publications India Pvt Ltd
B-42 Panchsheel Enclave
Post Box 4109
New Delhi 100 017

British Library Cataloguing in Publication data

A catalogue record for this book is available from the British Library

ISBN 0 7619 7144 0
ISBN 0 7619 7145 9 (pbk)

Library of Congress Control Number: 2003112191

Printed in India at Gopsons Papers Ltd, Noida

contents

acknowledgements

I am grateful to Karen Phillips for her help and encouragement in the early stages of getting this book off the ground; her faith in the project was very much appreciated. Thanks are also due to Alison Poyner for helpful discussions along the way and to Rachel Burrows for seeing the book through to press. The intensive care nurses who gave generously of their time and insights made this work possible; my thanks to them.

A number of friends and colleagues have given advice and comment and generally eased the production of this book. My thanks especially to Kenneth Boyd, Ken Mason, Alexander McCall Smith, Anne Murcott and Fran Wasoff. The island of Symi has also played its part in getting the words onto the page.

Lastly my thanks to the University of Edinburgh for sabbatical leave which made it possible to undertake the fieldwork, and to the ESRC for the Research Fellowship during which the book was completed.

i health care ethics

This book focuses on the empirical reality of clinical practice as a means of opening up ethical debates in health care. Whilst many publications take a moral philosophical approach to discussing the ethical debates which take place in health care practice, this book lays emphasis on the nature of the day to day practice of health care and so the ethical debates are presented in the context of the social organisation of health care practice. The book concentrates on intensive care. This is not because of a belief that it is only intensive care that gives rise to the hottest ethical debates, but rather because the fundamental issues which are typically debated in an intensive care context are also relevant across many areas of health care. This is in part because intensive care itself is not an entirely independent and separate entity; it has links and resonance with other areas of health care.

Given the central place which intensive care now occupies in hospital care, it is hard to remember that it has only been around since the mid twentieth century. Moreover, it is difficult to believe that its acceptance within medicine was slow to come about. The 1952 Copenhagen polio epidemic was the catastrophe which marked the birth of intensive care, as it was then that the centrality of the part that assisted ventilation played in the management of the critically ill was recognised. Le Fanu puts it well when he says:

> At any one time a patient can be hitched up to a dozen or more pieces of equipment: heart monitor, machines to measure the concentration of gases in the blood and the blood pressure, a pacemaker, a dialysis machine. It all looks, and is, so impressive that it can be difficult to appreciate that central to all this technological wizardry is just one piece of equipment, the ventilator blowing oxygen into the lungs. Oxygen alone ensures the heart carries on beating and 'buys time' for tissues to heal and the complications of impaired body function to be attended to. (1999: 72)

It was in the Copenhagen epidemic that teams of medical students were employed to hand ventilate the children with polio. Ironically it was the low regard in which anaesthetists were held which delayed there being the response to the lessons learned in Copenhagen. Le Fanu says that the view of the time regarding anaesthetists was that 'they were not really "proper doctors" but technicians whose competence did not stand beyond the operating theatre' (1999: 95).

Yet it was the transfer of thinking from the anaesthetics context to the needs of those patients dying from polio in 1952 which led to the development of the speciality of intensive care which still today centres on the capacity to artificially ventilate a patient. This slowness to recognise the contribution of anaesthetists to the speciality in which they now take the lead role is a good example of the importance of context in the practice of health care. In a discussion of how it was that ventilation was not used for other groups of patients who would clearly have benefited, such as those recovering from major surgery, Le Fanu concludes that:

> Many surgeons were ... implacably opposed to the proposal, fearing that post-operative ventilation could be interpreted as suggesting that 'something had gone wrong', which in turn might be construed as a reflection on their surgical competence. And so in the early 1950s patients who had been ventilated during major surgery such as open heart operations would be sent back to the ward 'breathing spontaneously', and as a result would develop a whole series of medical complications to which they would succumb. The mortality rate in the early days of cardiac surgery was as high as that for infantrymen at the Battle of the Somme, which has usually been attributed to the relative inexperience of surgeons in undertaking these innovative operations, but in reality is due to the fact that most of these patients were inadequately ventilated following the operation. (1999: 81)

Intensive care is heavily reliant upon the input of nursing: in fact, without the high ratio of nurses to patients intensive care does not exist. The definition of intensive care (Department of Health 1996) requires that each patient is cared for according to the ratio of one nurse to one patient and that there is a doctor present on the unit. This contrasts with high dependency nursing, where the ratio may be less than one nurse per patient and the doctor need only be on call. The Intensive Care Society (1997) recommendation is that each intensive care unit (ICU) bed requires seven whole time equivalent nursing posts. This provides twenty-four hour cover allowing for holidays and anticipated sick leave. The largest budget item in intensive care is the nursing salary bill.

Whatever may be the reality, there is a tendency to regard intensive care as the area within the hospital which has the concentration of ethical issues. It was after all the development of these areas of high tech medicine which was one of the reasons for ethical debate to come to the forefront of medicine. Once it became possible to maintain life by means of mechanical support whilst damaged organs recovered, the end of life became a far less certain entity and moral dilemmas came along with this uncertainty (Fox 1957). However the ethical issues which arise in the intensive care unit are in many ways the same as those which arise in any area of clinical practice: they have, among other things, to do with respect for persons and the balance between doing good and causing harm. Ethical issues may present in a stark form in the ICU, but it is often the case that such dilemmas carry lessons for other, less dramatic, occurrences in less acute settings.

Of course some of the ethical issues that arise in the ICU do so as a function of that setting, and by virtue of the condition of the patient. ICU patients are invariably vulnerable, very probably unconscious, and in any event not capable of conducting their own affairs. The ethical dimension of care, nursing or medical, is sufficiently fundamental to practice that it will often transcend the particular moral concerns which are directly driven by the setting. For instance, the question of autonomy and the fact that health care professionals are charged with acting in the best interests of patients, even when it is not clear what these are, will arise in various clinical settings when patients are for one reason or another not capable of directing their own affairs.

Nonetheless the ICU makes a useful place from which to start the examination of ethical issues because the nature of ICU work is such that ethical issues arise routinely. This book therefore draws upon the ethical issues which arise in intensive care as a starting point for arriving at general ethical ground rules for ethics in health care. The practices in the ICU are designed to meet the clinical needs of the patients who are admitted, but the effects of intensive care are more far-reaching. The existence of these intensive care practices and technologies causes a rise in expectations of provision in other areas of care which, to paraphrase the legal right to a hearing – our day in court – can give rise to a view that 'we all have a right to our day in intensive care'.

In this book I adopt the position which Beauchamp and Childress (1994; 2001) have put forward in relation to biomedical ethics debates. Beauchamp and Childress (1994; 2001) have written extensively about the *four ethical principles* which they argue can be employed in ethical debate, whatever the substantive issue in question. The principles are: respect for autonomy, non-maleficence, beneficence and justice (2001: 12). On this analysis, whilst the ethical issues and clinical cases may differ in detail, they maintain that the underlying ethical principles and positions are the same and for the most part can be traced back to the four principles.

Gillon says in praise of the four principles approach to practical ethics that it

offers a transcultural, transnational, transreligious, transphilo-
sophical framework for ethical analysis; that it offers elements of
a common language for such ethical analysis ... Because it is not
itself a theory, but instead draws on elements common to most if
not all moral theories, it can function peaceably as a tool of practical ethics that may be shared by those whose theories are totally
incompatible and antithetical. (1994: 332)

The intensive care setting tends to sharpen debate and the moral issue in
question often presents in terms of a dilemma. Whilst many of the moral
questions which arise in intensive care can also be found in other less
dramatic areas of health care, it is more likely to be the case that the
question of prolongation of life arises in the ICU. The question does arise
elsewhere, for example in care of the elderly facilities. However, since
the ICU is now such an important part of health care, and as intensive
care is increasingly looked to as a routinely available hospital facility, its
existence poses ethical questions for health care professionals and society as a whole. For these reasons, intensive care is taken in this book as
a starting point for the discussion of health care ethics. The premise of
the book is that it is instructive to examine the moral questions which
arise in intensive care in order to understand how moral decisions are
taken and how ethical issues are debated and handled in health care
more generally.

Beauchamp and Childress's four principles approach to bioethics
has come to occupy a central position, with defenders and detractors,
but nevertheless commanding a clear place in health care ethics debates
(Gillon and Lloyd 1994). This approach is essentially one which draws
upon moral philosophy or bioethics and so does rather leave out the
social context of the ethical problem, that is to say the organisational
issues, interpersonal factors, professional obligations and legal constraints. It is this contextual aspect of the moral dimension of care that is
addressed in this book.

This book sets out to bring a sociological analysis to a discussion of
some of the ethical issues encountered in health care. It is argued that the
combination of both sociological and philosophical perspectives assists
in our understanding of the moral dimension of health care practice. The
social organisation of health care practice is an important part of the
social context of care.

Before we turn to consider the nature of the literature on nursing
and medical ethics, some ground-laying work needs to be done to outline the substantive areas covered in the following chapters. In Chapter
2 the central concerns of intensive care are addressed: they include decisions around admission to the ICU and the continuation with or withdrawal of treatment.

Chapter 3 furthers the discussion of 'when to treat' and includes
debates about when aggressive treatment is appropriate or palliation

should be the course of action. Differences between nursing and medical perspectives are in sharp contrast in this discussion. The movement between care, cure and palliation has to be understood in the social context of public expectation, advances in technology and medical science, and questions of resources. Chapter 4 addresses the idea of caring for bodies and considers what relevance the sociology of the body literature has for health care ethics. This chapter includes a discussion of whether feeding by artificial means should be regarded as treatment and thereby be open to discontinuation when the prognosis is bad. Recent legal decisions are relevant here but we see that there remain difficulties in practice when professionals try to do what seems to be the right (moral) thing and at the same time have a concern for the legal and social implications of their actions.

The last chapter needs no detail here as it draws out the main arguments of the book which have already been outlined. The main argument of this final chapter demonstrates that it is important to locate ethical debates about health care in their clinical and social context in order to take account of the working practices and professional cultures of those involved. It concludes that intensive care provides a model for teamwork and consensus practice which can be generalised to other areas of health care where clinical decisions are difficult and interprofessional differences of opinion exist. These issues are often concerned with withdrawal of treatment at the end of life. There are other areas of practice where technological possibilities are morally fraught, examples being in paediatric intensive care, reproductive medicine and the care of the elderly. The lessons we can draw from intensive care have a place in the debates about the ethics in these other areas of health care.

INTENSIVE CARE AND THE HEALTH SERVICE

Intensive care is an area of clinical practice where teamwork is essential and one in which different professional cultures are brought into close proximity. One of the features of ethical debate in health care is the power relationship that exists between medicine and nursing: this is an important element in the working out of ethical questions. Intensive care, then, serves as an example of a clinical setting where we are likely to see teamwork in practice. Throughout the book I argue that intensive care has significance for those inside and outside its boundaries because its very existence gives rise to debates about how the end of life, or its prolongation, should be handled. The existence of intensive care and the fact that admission to an ICU is a possible course of action in the management of severe illness has an impact on our perceptions of what is possible. The ethical and financial issues which constrain intensive care practice are essentially to do with keeping sight of the criteria for admission. The central question of 'Should this patient be admitted to the ICU?' focuses upon the potential for a good outcome. If a patient is unlikely to benefit from intensive care it is not in his interests to spend time in the ICU, nor for that matter is it an ethical use of an expensive resource.

The ICU can be seen either as a microcosm of hospital care, a locale where the nature of the work makes teamwork paramount and moral consensus highly desirable, or it can be seen as a rather separatist elite area of practice which has problems of a different ethical order from the rest of health care. This latter view would suggest that the moral dimension of intensive care work is such that it has no relevance for other areas of health care. Throughout the book I argue for the former position: that is, intensive care represents a 'microcosm of hospital care' and as such can be the starting point for understanding ethical issues for health care. Ethical debates which start in the intensive care unit can be extrapolated to other areas of health care. And ethical ground rules which can be drawn up for intensive care can operate equally well in all areas of health care.

It is the case that for other areas of practice the existence of intensive care opens up the possibility of aggressive treatment which may offer short term benefits, yet in the long run such a course of action may not be in the best interests of many patients. Intensive care is a high profile aspect of health care and the public have high, often unrealistic, expectations of it. So whether intensive care is viewed from outside or from within the speciality, it can be said that the fact of its existence shapes the ethical debates in health care. These debates extend beyond the boundaries of intensive care and carry implications for practice in and beyond the ICU. Zussman (1992: 107), in his discussion of medical ethics and intensive care, cites a clinician who describes admission to an ICU as an 'escalation of the battle'. The view that intensive care is available as a possible line of treatment for all produces the situation alluded to above, where there is a culture which suggests the idea that every patient has a right to their 'day in an ICU', similar to the common-sense notion of a legal right to 'a day in court'.

The book draws lessons which can be applied more widely in health care from the discussion of ethical issues in intensive care. The book's theme is a concern with the way in which *nursing ethics* and *medical ethics* might better be played out as *health care ethics*. Essentially the argument here is that it would be a better idea to promote health care ethics, rather than continuing with the present parallel existence of medical ethics and nursing ethics literatures and debates. This formulation would put the patient in the centre and emphasise the importance of interdisciplinary teamwork in the health care system. Issues raised in clinical practice are complex and entail questions around professional teamwork, power relationships, hospital organisation, and ethical and legal considerations. Health care ethics would also be more suited to teamwork by virtue of being less adversarial. Nursing and medicine, the two main professional groups involved, could adopt less discipline-specific approaches to ethics in health care. Health care ethics would also be more in keeping with a multidisciplinary approach to care and with the realities of organisational life and clinical practice. The suggestion is that the two main professions in health care – medicine and nursing – should work towards a health care ethics, with a focus on patient need rather than professional interests.

The approach taken in the book is to bring together the sociological analysis of how the care is *actually* brought about and the moral philosophical perspective on what that care *should* entail. Medical and nursing ethics are concerned with such debates; both draw upon the arguments and theories of moral philosophers. A sociological analysis is helpful in allowing us to get a handle on how these two professional groups engage in and act upon these moral debates. In particular the sociological analysis will help to show that the old divisions of nursing and medical ethics are perhaps less relevant than they once were in the light of new forms of multiprofessional work practices. The main focus is upon the sociological analysis of clinical practice, which allows an examination of the social organisation of that practice. This provides an analysis of the context within which ethical issues arise and must be handled. The context is sometimes part of the problem and, of necessity, has to be considered in its resolution. Zussman (1992) is concerned with medical ethics, particularly with informed consent and decisions to withdraw treatment in the ICU. He argues for the sociological analysis because he says that medical ethics tends to concentrate on how decisions *should* be made and so misses out on how they *are* made in daily practice. Empirical work is important to gain this understanding of how decisions are made.

I start by drawing upon my work (Melia 2000a and b; 2001) which involved interviewing intensive care nurses and focused on the everyday clinical practice of intensive care in order to discuss the ethical issues that confronted ICU nurses in the course of their work.[1] The central concern of the study was to explore how, in a day to day sense, the often difficult, sometimes impossible situations which arise in ICUs are handled. By studying the practices, and the nurses' views on those practices, which form the work of intensive care I gained an understanding of how intensive care is accomplished. Such an approach also offers an insight into the costs – social, ethical and fiscal – of that accomplishment.

The major concern of the nurses in my study was with the limiting and withdrawal of treatment in cases where medical intervention and intensive care are deemed to be clinically and morally futile. This was the issue which was raised by the intensive care nurses when I asked about the ethically difficult aspects of their work. I did not set out specifically to study the withdrawal of treatment, but ended up with a study which focused on precisely that, as it is the crucial question for those, nurses and doctors, working in intensive care. The prime concern is to admit those who will benefit and to know when to stop when the benefit no longer is in prospect. This book is in large part concerned with that same issue, namely withholding and withdrawing intensive care.

I also draw extensively on the work of three authors publishing in the same field – Zussman (1992), Chambliss (1996) and Jennings (1986; 1990). These social scientists, in their different ways, have brought together a sociological analysis of the moral issues which emerge in the day to day practice of intensive care. Their work influenced my thinking and provides a platform from which to consider ethical issues within the context of the social organisation of clinical practice and of professional teamwork.

A number of social scientists studying the work of the medical profession, notably Fox (1989) and Zussman (1992), have argued that the social context is largely left out of discussions of medical ethics. Fox (1989: 229) noted that medical ethics writings often convey the idea that medical decisions are rational, contractual agreements made between individual patients and doctors with no recourse to the social context. In fact a closer examination of the empirical work available (Atkinson 1995; Chambliss 1996; Melia 2001; Seymour 2000; Zussman 1992) shows that the arrival at a decision about withdrawal of treatment is a social process which involves negotiation and discussion. It is not a matter of simply following ethical guidelines.

THE NATURE OF ETHICAL DEBATES IN INTENSIVE CARE

The standard way into debates on the ethical issues encountered in intensive care in medical or nursing ethics texts is to lay out the arguments and the options, giving structure to the issues by framing them within the theories of moral philosophy: typically these would be utilitarian, deontological, rights-based theory and so on. This leaves aside the social context of the actions in question.

Zussman (1992) argues that the social context must be taken into account and stresses that it is not the case that professionals can weigh up the philosophical arguments and reach a decision as if they were operating in a vacuum. The inclusion of a sociological analysis in the discussion of ethical issues provides some way out of this difficulty. Zussman states that: 'If sociology cannot tell us how matters of medical ethics should be resolved it can tell us how, in fact, they are resolved' (1992: 2).

Zussman argues that the power of medicine in decision making in relation to the difficult question of aggressive treatment is in decline in favour of the law. As patients' rights are increasingly being given prominence, Zussman argues, physicians are reserving decisions to themselves – decisions which they maintain are technical, not moral, in nature. As Zussman puts it:

> If physicians are prepared to acknowledge the rights of patients in the broad direction of medical care, they are also insistent on reserving some decisions to themselves as matters of technique. Families do not always agree. Thus, the lines of conflict are drawn. The point in question is not whether patients have rights. All agree that they do. Neither is the question whether those rights may be exercised on behalf of the patient by the patient's family. Most agree that they may. Rather, the issue becomes one of the limits of rights, of the boundary between matters of value and matters of technical knowledge. (1992: 97)

Chambliss (1996), in a study of intensive care, draws attention to the fact that nurses are in the position of implementing care and treatment without taking decisions on prognosis and the management of patients. This subordinated position of nursing relative to medicine, the occupation charged with making the decisions, he argues, is at the root of some of the ethical issues in ICUs. He notes, as does Zussman, that the power of medicine is being challenged by the prominence given to patients' rights and the increasing involvement of the law in what were traditionally medical decisions.

Chambliss maintains, however, that the ethical debates in intensive care often come about as a result of professional clashes. Interprofessional difficulties which stem from status differences between doctors and nurses have been well documented (Freidson 1970; Stein 1967). Negotiated order (Strauss 1978; Strauss et al. 1963) is perhaps the most useful analysis in the context of doctor–nurse interaction in the ICU. Mackay (1993) has noted that one central feature of negotiation between medicine and nursing is that there should be no disagreement in the presence of patients.

Chambliss argues that ethical problems are structurally created in the organisation, they are not individual, and they tend to arise when professional groups clash. It is when there is disagreement that the moral agendas are brought out by nurses who then seek to present the problem in ethical terms. In the work of Chambliss we see how different the sociological analysis is from the philosophical approach. The sociological analysis points up the context in which these ethical questions are resolved and shows that, in addition to the ethical principles which shape the moral questions, the organisational and social contexts are important. Empirical work presented in later chapters demonstrates the importance of context. Just as Zussman (1992) has given us an insight into the workings of medicine when ethical issues arise, Chambliss

(1996) offers a sociological analysis of nursing ethics, and presents what he calls the 'social organisation of ethics'. On this view, nursing ethics is often more a manifestation of the power struggles between the two occupational groups, with nursing, the less powerful, resorting to moral argument as a means of achieving some control.

Jennings (1990: 222) has made the point that sociology and moral philosophy have something to offer each other when it comes to explaining moral difficulties that are inherent in health care. He argues that new-born intensive care is a particularly good subject for exploring the general difficulties – as well as the potential benefits – of forging a closer connection between ethnography and ethics. Jennings (1990: 223) noted that in the neonatal intensive care unit much of the ethical discussion was focused on the decision making process in relation to life-sustaining treatment. The 'best interest' standard was followed when quality of life decisions were being made. He concludes that ethnographic studies of life within neonatal intensive care units (NICUs) should provide telling information about how decisions are made and why. He says that studies of NICUs can point the way to what he calls 'ethically preferred decision-making processes', but that they will also draw attention to 'some of the subtle costs and cultural consequences' of the changes in practice. Jennings's analysis shows that the technological imperative is strong in the NICU and that erring on the side of over-treatment is commonplace in order that the potential risk of under-treating is minimised. His work can be regarded as seminal for those interested in the sociological analysis of the clinical settings in which moral decisions are taken and where such decisions are an integral part of daily practice.

The work of Jennings (1990) with its emphasis on the contributions that moral philosophy and sociology can make to the study of ethics in neonatal intensive care influenced my work on the ethical issues in intensive care nursing (Melia 2001).[2] The approach to obtaining and analysing the data was sociological. As Jennings puts it: 'as ethics by definition involves human relations and human doings, all work in ethics makes nearly constant reference to behavioral, psychological and social description' (1990: 221).

Jennings has written widely on the theme of the relationship of social science and ethics in the context of applied ethics and policy analysis. In his paper 'Applied ethics and the vocation of social science', he suggests that

> disciplinary boundaries separating ethics from social science have begun to blur and break down … like geological plates shifting to overlap in new ways, descriptive social scientific analysis appears to be increasingly value-laden while normative ethical analysis becomes increasingly fact-laden. Applied studies in ethics are one fault line where the shifts are most evident and potentially most significant in their consequences. (1986: 207)

The thrust of Jennings's argument is that studies of applied and professional ethics constitute more than just another subdivision within academic philosophy. Those philosophers who work in the area of applied ethics, Jennings says, occupy a rather uncomfortable middle ground between the theoretical rigour of their academic discipline and the day to day experience involving practical judgement of the professional and the political worlds that they seek to influence (1986: 209).

The literature on nursing ethics is extensive and could also be subjected to Jennings's critique of medical ethics in so far as it tends to focus on discussions of cases which are designed to illustrate the various ethical theories and positions of philosophers whose writings are traditionally drawn upon in medical and nursing ethics: Aristotle (trans. 1976), Kant (1788), Mill (1861) and Rawls (1972). These medical and nursing ethics texts have their place, but as health care professionals become increasingly familiar with this kind of debate, they question how good is the fit between this literature and the clinical practice it serves. Also there are ongoing debates among philosophers and practitioners concerning the utility of medical ethics.

SOCIOLOGICAL AND PHILOSOPHICAL APPROACHES TO ETHICAL ISSUES

The approach I have taken in this book assumes that ethical debates within intensive care nursing might benefit from a sociological treatment. In a paper addressing the 'Task of nursing ethics' (Melia 1994) I have argued that historically there has been a lack of empirical work in nursing ethics and that this has led to a perpetuation of the tendency to examine ethical issues in a rather stylised way, whereby the work of a few philosophers is routinely used as the vehicle through which to discuss ethical issues in health care. This approach is not without its merits: however the resultant analysis can be said to suffer from a lack of context. Jennings's (1986; 1990) work in neonatal intensive care offers a clear case for combining the moral philosophical and the sociological approach to the study of applied professional ethics. Moral philosophers tend to move back and forth between individual illustrative cases and their theoretical propositions and ethical principles, whereas sociologists are attempting to understand the situation as it is and will therefore tend to have some empirical basis to their studies. It is really too much of a caricature to say that philosophers are interested in data (cases) only in so far as they illustrate their arguments, just as it will not do to say that sociologists dismiss ethical debate as someone else's business, rather than taking it on as a serious part of their enterprise. Yet, there is a grain of truth in these caricatures. The moral philosophical and the sociological approach to the study of health care when there is a moral dimension to the work differ probably in emphasis more than anything and so we should not hesitate to combine the two if a more useful analysis results.

One of the main differences in approach between the social scientist and moral philosopher is that ethical theories tend to hold that human beings are capable of rational, responsible, autonomous behaviour and so talk of moral agency, personhood, autonomy and so on. Social science, on the other hand, Jennings (1986) argues, developed theoretical perspectives which were at odds with those traditionally employed in ethical theory. Social science produced a set of categories which focused on the more structural and external influences upon human behaviour (1986: 215–16). These social-science-driven ways of seeing the world and the place of the individual within it which have developed in response to the rise of the bureaucratic nation state have, according to Jennings, led to a move away from the framework of ethical theory in our attempts to understand the world. Jennings, writing in the late 1980s, says that the climate in social science has changed since the 1970s in such a way as to become a good deal more receptive to the traditional categories of moral agency. He puts this down to the rise of interpretive methods in social science research. Jennings is suggesting not that interpretive methods have replaced the deterministic explanation of the social world, but that they have, as he puts it, 'mitigated the extremism of that vision' (1986: 216). With less emphasis upon behaviourism and positivism, he argues, there is scope for the older categories of autonomy and responsibility to have their place. As research in health care and in nursing in particular has adopted qualitative, interpretive methods with some enthusiasm, Jennings's position is especially apposite. It could also be argued that the move in health care towards an open and accountable service delivery makes Jennings's point about the place of ideas to do with autonomy and reason increasingly relevant.

Jennings (1990) compares two analyses of neonatal intensive care units. One is the work of an ethicist, the other that of an ethnographer. Their perspectives are so different that the result appears as if different subject matter had been the subject of study. Jennings notes that the stock explanation for the discrepancy is that 'ethnographers are talking about the world of neonatology as it is and ethicists are talking about neonatology as it should be' (Jennings 1990: 226).

This explanation, Jennings says, is inadequate, not least because as most ethicists have some experience of neonatal intensive care they are not only talking of the 'oughts'. Also, ethnographers may not overtly or explicitly express their views on the desired *modus operandi* in an intensive care unit, but their emphasis in analysis is upon the importance of shared communication among professionals and parents; this has ethical implications as well as sociological force. Jennings argues that moral philosophers take as given the capacity to perceive issues as moral issues and to understand and use moral concepts and categories. According to

Jennings philosophers do not see

> moral concepts and categories as embedded in ongoing forms of
> social practice and experience that are structured via particular
> institutional patterns or the encounter with certain technological
> constraints.

Nor do they

> pay much attention to the ways in which struggling with a prob-
> lem or acting within a certain pattern of constraints or power rela-
> tionships can actually transform the moral perception and under-
> standing of agents. (1990: 229)

Both Zussman (1992) and Chambliss (1996) have also paid attention to
these issues, and in my study of intensive care ethics (Melia 2001) I took
heed of their exhortation to examine ethical issues in their social context.
By means of detailed qualitative interviews insights were gained into the
ways in which some of the most contentious decisions are taken and carried through in the clinical setting. The bringing together of sociological
analysis and philosophical insights serves to demonstrate how the moral
questions in health care are embedded in daily social practices. The
moral issues cause practitioners to question their everyday practices. At
the same time the sociological analysis shows that everyday practices
serve, to some extent, to buffer and routinise the moral aspects of care.

This need for an analysis of the context within which ethical decisions are made is recognised by some writers in medical ethics, and their
solution is to take what they describe as a narrative ethics approach
(Brody 1994). Brody puts it well when he says:

> my own work as an ethics consultant and as a member of a hos-
> pital ethics committee has caused me to join similarly placed col-
> leagues in finding that formal methods of ethical reasoning
> describe very poorly our actual day-to-day practices. (1994: 207)

Narrative ethics, like casuistry, seeks to include context and care analysis rather than rely too heavily on formal moral philosophical style of
debate and argumentation. The social context is important here because
much of the day to day practice of intensive care has to do with effecting
clinical possibilities in socially acceptable ways. The analysis of the context and ways in which the ethical decisions are taken illustrates how the
'socially acceptable' is important if we are to understand the moral
dimension of care.

This book is informed by the idea that advances in medical science
and technology, along with the high expectations of an informed and
educated society, have rendered the concept of 'end of life' problematic.
Intensive care units accept patients in a range of clinical circumstances

mostly involving organ failure; the need which these patients have in common is life support and intensive nursing care. The fact that the ICU raises possibilities for care and treatment when the outlook is poor means that questions about how the end of life is managed or prolonged are moral issues for those working in intensive care.

The ethical issues which the development of intensive care has brought with it, or at least contributed to, are considered in this book. The advances in intensive care provision raise questions about when it is reasonable to adopt aggressive treatment. The concept of futility in connection with medical intervention is not a clear-cut entity. Wider questions of quality of life, the duty of care, informed consent and resource allocation are involved. These are clinical, moral and legal issues which have to be considered by those managing the care of patients in these 'end of life' situations and in circumstances where intensive care is a problematic option. Neonatal intensive care is an obvious example of an area where what might be called 'heroic treatment' presents moral dilemmas for those involved.

Unlike many medical or nursing ethics texts, in this book I draw upon empirical data which would be more at home in a sociological work. The contributions of moral philosophical insights and sociological analysis allow an examination of clinical practice in the context of professional cultures and everyday work situations. I argue throughout that the separatist configuration of medical ethics and nursing ethics has served to perpetuate the differences that exist between the two professions, rather than to mediate them and to suggest ways of interprofessional co-operation. The work drawn upon demonstrates that there is a social organisation of clinical practice which involves the different professional groups working together in teams, and in so doing coming to discuss the ethical dimension of practice in the context of that multiprofessional team. The lessons from the intensive care setting, where teamwork is a *sine qua non*, can be translated to other areas of practice. We can draw from the analysis of day to day practice in intensive care and begin to lay down the general ground rules for ethical practice which are common to all professional groups concerned.

MEDICAL ETHICS AND NURSING ETHICS

We can now turn to a consideration of the nature of the literature on nursing and medical ethics. The intention is not to present a conventional review of the medical and nursing ethics literatures, but rather to characterise the essence of these literatures and to use this as a basis from which to argue for abandoning the traditional professional fault lines and instead make the case, as stated above, for health care ethics.

The ethical debates as they have developed and been published in the literature of medicine and nursing are similar in many ways.

Common to both nursing and medical ethics texts is the presentation of a range of ethical theories which are thought to be useful as the framework within which to discuss the ethical questions that arise in health care. Both follow a standard cast list of philosophers and present the arguments of different moral philosophical positions: utilitarianism, deontological, rights-based ethics, virtue ethics and so on. The model set by medicine was followed by nursing to a large extent. The arguments put forward for the need for a nursing ethics literature which is separate from medical ethics usually run along the lines that the nursing experience is different from the medical one in any given case by virtue of the different nature of their roles *vis-à-vis* diagnosis, prescription and the management of the patient.

A considerable body of literature now comes under the nursing ethics heading. This started at the beginning of the twentieth century in the United States, with a good deal being written in the first twenty years or so; this tailed off in the 1940s and 1950s. However, from the 1970s onwards there has been a steady rise in the production of nursing ethics texts and journal articles on the subject. Some of this growth can perhaps be attributed to the expansion of academic nursing, but it is nevertheless the case that the moral dimension of health care has come firmly onto the agenda for both nursing and medicine.

This interest in the moral dimension of health care and in professional ethics has, of course, come about in response to the possibilities that medical science has opened up for health care. Important too is the fact that we are now a more informed and educated society with higher expectations. Mason (1988), in his discussion of the dramatic changes that have come about in medicine since the Second World War, points to paediatrics as an area where the notion of *quality of life* as opposed to *life at all costs* began to take hold. Since then we have witnessed similar debates each time a scientific advance opens up new possibilities: life support, organ transplantation, genetic screening and manipulation and so on. Mason describes as a 'remarkable shift from the Hippocratic position' the move which he says medicine has made 'towards an ethos which was influenced by the concept of preserving the *quality* of life rather than of endowing life with an absolute value' (1988: 4, my emphasis).

The ethics literature of both professional groups, medicine and nursing, focuses on professional codes of ethics and quite properly concentrates on debates about the ethical basis of their practice. Medical ethics texts tend to concentrate on how ethical decisions should be made. The nursing literature has questioned this focus on medical activity and followed two different approaches to ethical debates which are thought to be more appropriate for nurses. The first centres around the idea of nurses taking on the role of patient's advocate. The second approach has resulted in the proliferation of a literature concerned with the 'ethic of care'. We will return later in the chapter to these approaches taken up by nursing.

DEDUCTIVE REASONING

Deductive reasoning, from the general theory or principle to the particular case, with the former giving direction for the action in the latter, is a common approach to biomedical ethics. Beauchamp and Childress (1994; 2001) argue that reasoning in an inductive way, starting with existing social practices and generalising to norms and rules, is an equally plausible method of relating ethical theory to moral judgements. In Beauchamp and Childress's words:

> Inductivists ... argue that we reason inductively from particular instances to general statements or positions. Inductivists hold that we use existing social agreements and practices, insight-producing novel cases, and comparative case analysis as the initial starting point from which to make decisions in particular cases and to generalize to norms. Inductivists emphasize an evolving moral life that reflects exemplary lives and narratives, experience with hard cases and analogy from prior practice. (2001: 391)

One reason for concentrating heavily on Beauchamp and Childress in this account is that they give a clear view on the different kinds of justification and, importantly, they acknowledge the fact that moral theories should not be too readily pigeon-holed, as proponents of one theory do not necessarily disregard other methods in their moral reasoning (1994: 19). Having examined the deductive and inductive modes, they point out that there are shortcomings to be found in both approaches and offer a third alternative which they term *coherence theory*, which is neither an inductive nor a deductive approach but one which moves in both directions. In their words:

> 'The top' (principles, theories) and 'the bottom' (cases, individual judgements) are not solely sufficient for biomedical ethics. Neither general principles nor paradigm cases have sufficient power to generate conclusions with the needed reliability. Principles need to be made specific for cases, and case analysis needs illumination from general principles. (2001: 397)

The four principles approach represents Beauchamp and Childress's ethical framework for the discussion and debate of the moral issues which arise in medical practice. They recognise that

> although rules, rights and virtues are of the highest importance for health care ethics, principles provide the most abstract and comprehensive norms in the framework. (1994: 37)

The four principles derive from accepted moral positions, from 'considered judgements', a term used by Rawls (1972) in *A theory of justice*, and medical tradition. Beauchamp and Childress state that they only make a 'loose distinction' between rules and principles, but hold that

> principles do not function as precise action guides that inform us in each circumstance how to act in the way that more detailed rules do. Principles are more general guides that leave considerable room for judgement in specific cases and that provide substantive guidance for the development of more detailed rules and policies. (1994: 38)

I have sketched the arguments of Beauchamp and Childress here, drawing on their chapters on 'moral theories' and 'method and moral justification'. Their purpose is to give a wider account of moral reasoning than offered by what they regard as the more restricted idea of 'applied ethics'. It is interesting to note, in the context of the main theme of this book, that they say that they have, in their words, 'hinted at an interdisciplinary account of biomedical ethics' (1994: 40).

As I have noted earlier in this chapter, it is not the intention here to provide a comprehensive account of the literatures of medical and nursing ethics; rather it is to present a characterisation of them which represents their essential nature. My purpose is to point to the possible alternative, namely *health care ethics*, and to bring to bear on these ethical debates a sociological analysis of health care practices and moral philosophical insights.

In their introduction to the types of ethical theory, Beauchamp and Childress (1994; 2001) note a number of conditions which they deem to be necessary for ethical theory to be adequate. These include clarity, coherence, competence, comprehensiveness, simplicity, explanatory power, justificatory power and practicability. Demands made of theory are clearly not simple. However, if one becomes overwhelmed by conditions required for a workable theory for ethical debate then the utility of practical ethics begins to wane. I am not arguing for overly simplistic theory, as there comes a point where it can be so simplistic as to be not worth bothering with. However, among the conditions that Beauchamp and Childress set for adequate ethical theory I would give some prominence to clarity, practicability and explanatory power, recognising that this is no small order. There follows a brief account of the theories rehearsed in the literature of medical and nursing ethics.

UTILITARIANISM

Among the oft used theories in medical and nursing ethics texts is the consequence-based theory of Jeremy Bentham (1748–1832) and John

Stuart Mill (1806–1873), which centres on the idea of the greatest good for the greatest number. One important aspect of this approach to ethics is the consequence of actions. At its simplest a utilitarian theory would hold that an action was right or wrong as judged by the good or bad consequences yielded. The basic principle in operation here, as the name implies, is utility. In this connection Campbell (1984) has usefully noted that the problem for ethics in health care is that consequences are not always predictable. Taking up his point I would add that social context or a sociological commentary upon the circumstances in which a moral issue arises will not of course produce the answer to the problem of prediction; it will however go some way towards consideration of the total situation.

Within utilitarianism, in its original formulation, the central idea was that of the greatest happiness. The notion of utility, common good or benefit of the majority came with Mill's refinements of the theory, and it is this idea which has found its appeal in medical and nursing ethics (Campbell 1984). Some writers (Frankena 1973) distinguish between 'act' and 'rule' utilitarianism. Act utilitarianism focuses on the consequences of particular acts, whereas rule utilitarianism would focus on the following of a general rule as the best way to lead to the most desirable outcome for all concerned, that is the greatest number. Rule following in this way may not always lead to the greatest good, but the idea is that on balance to follow rules will lead on most occasions to the best outcome in terms of a utilitarian calculation.

As Beauchamp and Childress put it:

> the act utilitarian asks 'what good and bad consequences will result from *this action in this circumstance*?' For the act utilitarian, moral rules are useful in guiding human actions, but are also expendable if they do not promote utility in a particular context. For the rule utilitarian, by contrast, an act's conformity to a justified rule (that is, a rule justified by utility) makes the act right, and the rule is not expendable in a particular context, even if following the rule in that context does not maximize utility. (2001: 344)

One of the problems inherent with ethical theories is that each one has its strengths and its limitations; none covers all moral eventualities. The next type of theory stands in marked contrast to utilitarianism.

KANTIANISM: OBLIGATION-BASED THEORY

Deontological theory is another name for this theory, from the Greek *deon* meaning 'duty'. The Kantian label derives from its main author, the German philosopher Immanuel Kant (1724–1804). Campbell sums up the Kantian approach in words of which he says Kant would scarcely have approved:

> [Kant] believed that the guts of morality were to be found in the experience of doing one's duty for duty's sake and for no other reason. (1984: 74)

A more conventional definition of deontological theory is

> a general approach to the justification of ethical behaviour in which priority is given to fundamental principles, rights and duties. (Thompson et al. 2000: 364)

Kantian ethical theory is based, then, on the idea that it is the intended good that should come from doing one's duty that settles the question of rightness or wrongness of an action, not the actual consequences of an action. For Kant there were important features for a moral principle to be binding as a duty. It had to be universal, unconditional and imperative; that is, actions should or should not be done according to these criteria. Kant's idea of the categorical imperative comes from this line of argument. Campbell sums up the position when he says:

> if any particular maxim is proposed, it can only be accepted as a genuinely moral rule if it fulfils all the conditions laid down – universally applicable, coherent with a rational system of nature, capable of being freely adopted by a community of rational beings. (1984: 75)

In Kant's words, 'I ought never to act except in such a way that I can also will that my maxim become a universal law', and 'One must act to treat every person as an end and never as a means only.'

Kant believed that human beings were autonomous, rational beings who are capable of reasoning. Also that individuals have moral worth which makes it necessary for us to treat others as we would have them treat us. This principle of reciprocity is by no means peculiar to Kant, as this 'do as you would be done by' maxim is common to many philosophical positions. The idea that Kant is perhaps more closely associated with than any other philosopher is the notion that however worthy the intentions and expected outcome of an action, people must be treated as *ends in themselves* and not as *mere means to an end*. The old adage 'the ends justify the means' could not be further from this position. Kant's principle of 'respect for persons' is central to many debates in health care ethics, yet it leaves us with some difficult questions in health care. For instance, do some patients have less right to our respect because they are not 'rational beings'? Making the individual central to the argument is as difficult in its way as is trying to deal in quantification of the greatest good.

RIGHTS-BASED ETHICAL THEORY

It has become a commonplace to discuss health care in the language of rights: rights to treatment, privacy, choice and so on. Rights appeal to our libertarian instincts, but they are a complex matter, as they are neither clear-cut nor absolute. Beauchamp and Childress (2001: 356) describe rights in terms of 'liberal individualism', a situation which exists within democracies and which allows individuals to conduct themselves with a certain freedom, constrained only in so far as consideration of the rights of others must be taken into account: there are rules and laws which govern such democracies.

Rights are perhaps best thought of as justifiable claims, legal or moral, that individuals can make upon others or upon society. Rights usually correlate with duties. They can also conflict: my claim to something may conflict with another's right not to provide it. Legal rights are claims which are justified by recourse to the law, whereas moral rights are claims that are justified in terms of moral principles and rules.

Rights can be positive, for example to be provided with some benefit or service, or they can be negative, for example when a person can demand that someone desists from doing them harm or causing inconvenience. In discussing the limitations of a rights-based ethical theory, Beauchamp and Childress say that it should be understood not 'as a comprehensive or complete moral theory, but rather as an account of the minimal and enforceable rules that communities and individuals must observe in their treatment of all persons' (1994: 76).

CASUISTRY: APPLYING THEORY TO CASES

I include casuistry not because it is written about widely in the standard medical and nursing ethics texts, but because it carries with it some similarity with the sociological concern for including context in understanding behaviour in clinical practice. It is also close to narrative ethics. A further reason for its inclusion is that the main protagonists, Jonsen and Toulmin (1988; Jonsen 1995), have in the process of rehabilitating casuistry done some damage to the four principles approach, or at least such is the view of Beauchamp and Childress (2001: 393).

The idea of casuistry was influential in the Middle Ages but, as Thompson et al. note,

> it acquired a derogatory meaning at the time of the reformation when thinkers as different as Pascal and Luther criticised the Church for abandoning strict ethical principles, by applying the precedents and particular cases and 'practical ethics' to justify making all sorts of compromises with the absolute demands of the gospel. (2000: 98)

Beauchamp and Childress say that 'Casuistry refers to the use of case comparison and analogy to reach moral conclusions' (2001: 392). They go on to say that Jonsen and Toulmin (1988), in their rehabilitation of casuistry, 'spearheaded this approach to method in contemporary bio-medical ethics ... [and] have, in the process, criticised our framework of principles' (2001: 393).

Casuists are suspicious of rules and general theories which stand apart from cases or particular contexts and circumstances. Beauchamp and Childress state that casuists would argue that appropriate moral judgements are made through 'an intimate acquaintance with particular situations and the historical record of similar cases' (2001: 393). Toulmin (1981) has written of the 'tyranny of principles' when there is inflexibility and no account taken of context. Beauchamp and Childress note that casuists do not always ignore rules and principles in their moral thinking, but do 'insist that moral judgements can be and often are made when no appeal to principle is possible' (2001: 394). Casuistry is defended by Jonsen and Toulmin (1988) on the grounds that it produces agreement. Beauchamp and Childress put it neatly when they say: 'Moral certitude, then, is found at the bottom – in the case and traditions of practical judgement – not at the top in a principle or theoretical judgement' (2001: 393).

Gillon makes this useful comment on casuistry in one of his contributions to the tome which he edited with Lloyd:

> Casuistry is then the application of general ethical principles to particular cases. Under a different guise this is also the basis of the case law approach to English law. The four principles as a set of general *prima facie* moral principles are entirely compatible with casuistry which seeks to apply them to particular cases. (1994: 327)

VIRTUE ETHICS

Virtue ethics is one moral theory which is, following the work of MacIntyre (1981), gaining popularity in the texts on medical and nursing ethics. Campbell et al. best sum up virtue ethics when they say:

> According to virtue theory, it is character that is the focus of moral concern, and someone who shows virtues such as kindness, generosity, respect for persons, honesty, compassion and so forth will be the model of moral conduct. (1997: 7)

Clearly, the virtue ethics approach is more than leaving the question of ethics to the good sense and judgement of professionals. This is not to say that we should be naturally suspicious of health care professionals, for as Campbell et al. say, 'even the most vitriolic critics of doctors would accept that most are decent people acting as best they can according to their own lights' (1997: 7). They argue that what is needed is 'to devise a conception of virtuous practice that does not suggest that a doctor, for instance, can dictate what ought to happen to other people' (1997: 7).

In an earlier work, Campbell (1984) introduces the ethical theories employed in the discussion of medical ethics by moving from the more subjective, individual conscience-based theories to the more objective approaches of utilitarianism, natural law and theories based on respect for persons. Throughout his discussion of the various theories Campbell makes it clear that there is no ultimate ethical theory which will please all and cover all eventualities. This is a common theme in medical and nursing ethics texts: the point frequently made is that however limited they are these theories provide a framework and language for debating the ethical issues which arise in health care. There is an understandable attraction to the more 'objective' approaches as a move away from individual conscience makes societal debate and professional ethics more feasible. Campbell puts it well when he says, of what he calls 'the "plain man's" feeling that his conscience knows best' approach, 'we might say that such a view seems sensible enough until we meet two plain men who disagree' (1984: 36).

Virtue ethics perhaps offers some middle ground between the hopelessly subjective and the less useful abstract objectivity of some moral theories. Virtue ethics has been given prominence recently in ethics texts. MacIntyre in *After virtue* (1981) offers an alternative to the polarised, utilitarian versus deontological way in which ethical theory is often presented. The problem with the polarisation is that it suggests that it has to be one or the other. Virtue ethics focuses on the competence and integrity of the moral agent. As Thompson et al. put it, 'virtue ethics is as old as Aristotle (384–322 BC) and as new as MacIntyre's (1981) defence of virtue ethics' (2000: 303).

Thompson et al. say that what MacIntyre does in *After virtue* is to 'focus attention back onto the moral agent rather than the abstract principles, rights and duties on which we base our judgements or on the practical consequences or outcomes of our actions' (2000: 303). The problem often voiced in relation to utilitarianism and deontological theories is that they leave out the individual making the judgement and the social context in which the judgement is made. Virtue ethics remedies this by, in the words of Thompson et al., concentrating 'on the moral agent as the person who is responsible for deciding how to apply general moral principles to specific situations in order to bring about the desired consequences' (2000: 303).

Virtue ethics brings to our attention the fact that the quality of the action depends upon the integrity and competence of the moral agent.

Thompson et al. note that Aristotle, 'in his *Nicomachean ethics*, develops a system requiring two kinds of complementary skill or competency necessary for the balanced moral agent' (2000: 303).[3] These are the intellectual and the moral virtues. The intellectual, or theoretical, virtues include relevant scientific knowledge, technical skill and experience, intelligence, discriminatory judgement and practical wisdom. Aristotle's list of moral, or practical, virtues includes honesty, temperance, courage, justice, fairness and generosity. In some ways virtue ethics, with its focus on the attributes of the moral agent, is in danger of taking us back into the difficulties thrown up by reliance upon individual consciences for a guide to action. Campbell et al.'s (1997) call for a 'conception of virtuous practice' is the suggested way forward on this.

There is a current emphasis upon competency-based training in the health care professions; this is not without its difficulties. However there are, as Thompson et al. point out, clear links between virtue ethics and competence, and thus there is a particular relevance of virtue ethics for practice. They note that 'recent stress on "competencies", and attempts to define these, involve a return to something like the classical meaning of "virtue" as "proficiency or excellence in performance" and "vice" as "culpable incompetence"' (2000: 66).

ETHIC OF CARE AND ADVOCACY

The medical and nursing texts concerned with ethics follow in various ways an essentially similar pattern of presenting these different ethical theories including all or some of those outlined above. Cases and moral dilemmas are discussed in the light of these theories and the general principles that are associated with them. Whatever theory is chosen, there turns out to be a lack in some direction. The focus on the greatest number in utilitarianism leaves the individual or minority group out of the picture. The social and organisational context is also left out of the ethical debate on clinical practice if theory and principles are closely adhered to in a strictly moral philosophical style of argument. The relationships between the professions in health care, especially the power dimension to those relationships, are factors which enter into ethical debate. For nurses, ethical issues are often bound up with the organisational and managerial facts of the matter. It is therefore the case that the ways in which care is organised, and the nature of the working relationships between the different professional groups and between professionals and health care managers, have a bearing upon the ethical decisions that are made.

Whilst it is true to say that nursing and medical ethics texts follow a similar pattern, there are nonetheless differences in emphasis. Medical ethics is primarily concerned with decision making. Zussman (1992) argues that medical ethics has been fairly consistent in ignoring the social context in which medical decisions are made. As he puts it, 'Medical ethics, in short, has failed to acknowledge that everything in the contract is not contractual' (1992: 2). Also, despite the development of teamworking in health care, it remains a legal fact that it is the medical member of the team that carries the can for the decisions taken about diagnosis, treatment and management of the patient. All professionals are responsible for their actions and these are regulated by the appropriate professional regulatory procedures.

Perhaps because there is some recognition, implicit if not often stated, that at law responsibility for the decisions concerning management of care lies with medicine, nursing ethics texts have followed two particular themes which medical ethics texts were not dealing with. These are the *ethics of care* and *advocacy*. The ethics of care focuses on the activity of caring for people and addresses the issues which arise in that intimate person to person situation. Campbell et al. say that, 'the ethics of care focuses on the moral perceptions, dispositions and thoughts that arise from the actual business of caring for people' (1997: 14). They also note that:

> it [ethics of care] has grown up in nursing ethics where the problems of power hierarchies, the role of women, and the actual experience of tending to people's needs have combined to yield a very different perspective on the ethical situation from that traditionally found in books of medical ethics. (1997: 14)

Interestingly, Campbell et al. note the similarity of the ethics of caring and virtue ethics, and this is best offered in their words:

> In some ways it is a virtue theory, which emphasises the moral importance and insight of lived experience in the development of a caring character. What it has added is not a mere substitution of the concept of care for concepts like autonomy and beneficence, but rather a sensitive appreciation of practical needs, caring responses to those needs and the wisdom resulting from such encounters. (1997: 14)

The ethic of care, or certainly its popularity, owes much to the work of Carol Gilligan. Her book *In a different voice* (1982) presented a challenge to Kohlberg's (1976) analysis of moral reasoning by suggesting that there were gendered differences in approach to moral reasoning. In her analysis of girls' moral reasoning processes, Gilligan (1977) offered an ethic of care which she contrasted with the ethic of justice and rights – which was the model that Kohlberg argued boys in his study used in arriving at moral judgements. In 1993 Gilligan, in a comment on reactions to her earlier work, argued that she had been misrepresented by many who take the gender thesis too far and too literally. The 'different voice,' she notes, 'is identified not by gender but by theme'. She describes two

moral perspectives, care and justice, that, she says, 'organize both thinking and feelings and empower the self to take different kinds of action in
public as well as private life'. She says that the title of her book was
deliberate: it reads, she reminds us, *In a different voice*, not *In a woman's
voice* (1993: 209).

Ethics of care links to virtue ethics as it focuses on the activity of caring and therefore on the patient–professional relationship and so on the
moral agent. Writers in nursing ethics seized on Gilligan's work as a useful means of furthering nursing's professionalising project. At that time
nursing was interested in staking out and developing a distinctive role,
which would be different from that of medicine. Nursing's legacy of
being in a subordinate relationship to a dominant medical profession
adds further impetus to the desire by nurses to articulate a unique body
of knowledge for nursing and to develop an area of practice which nursing can claim as its own. In other words, nursing is engaged in the activity described by Hughes (1958) as the typical approach taken by an occupation striving to attain professional status. Among the hallmarks of a
profession is the possession of a code of professional ethics. It is clear,
then, that the debates which are central to nursing practice will also be
central to nursing's ethical debates.

Nursing has a particular relationship with medicine in the organisational structure of health care, and indeed in the hierarchy of occupa-
tions (Freidson 1970; Mackay 1993; Witz 1992). Whilst some aspects of
nursing are independent of medicine, it is in part dependent on the
diagnosis and treatment decisions of medicine. Nursing is therefore
keen to ring fence some activities as the particular domain of nursing.
By contrast, medicine is under some pressure to move away from the
position of the dominant profession in health care and to develop more
team-oriented approaches to health care. A series of recent events and
reports alongside the whole modernising project in the NHS is a further impetus to change in the social organisation of medical practice
(Department of Health 1997).

In so far as any occupation can claim autonomous professional status when working within a bureaucracy such as a nationalised health
care system, medicine has managed to lay claim to and maintain professional status in that it has control of its work and membership (Freidson
1970). As nursing work is dependent in part on medical practice, it is less
easy for nursing to make the same claims to autonomous professional
status. This dependency upon medicine means that nursing, when it
wishes to develop itself, has a tendency to want to pull away from medicine and engage in uniquely nursing activities and debates (Melia 1994).
In this regard, advocacy is the other theme taken up by nursing ethics
texts; this is not a feature of their medical counterparts. This focus on
advocacy adopts the position that the nurse is well placed to be the
patient's advocate. At first sight this seems to be a perfectly laudable

viewpoint: patients can be assured that their rights will be protected and their interests best served. However, upon further reflection it seems to me that the argument is flawed. The main difficulty is that advocacy has adversarial connotations. There is no reason to suppose that the nurse can be sufficiently removed from the ideology and organisation of health care, and from nursing's own ideology, to make and plead a patient's case as an advocate would be obliged to do. Also, it may bring a nurse into conflict with the duty of care, should the patient wish to do something that would not be in their best interests.

The balance of the patient's right to self-determination and the nurse's obligation to do the best for them in line with the duty of care is difficult enough to bring off at the best of times without the added complication of the nurse claiming to be the advocate. Nurses have power by virtue of their familiarity with the system, whereas patients are by and large vulnerable. So, at best, the activity of the nurse as advocate is likely to resemble benevolent paternalism on the part of the nurse, with the patient taking a passive trusting role. The charge of paternalism is usually levelled at medicine; however the nurse as advocate would produce a similar situation in those circumstances where the patient's wishes and the nurse's view of appropriate care did not coincide. It seems to me that Henderson's (1964) idea of doing for patients that which they cannot do for themselves more than covers what is really meant by the nurse as advocate, without confusing the issue by importing this legal terminology. It is also the case that when advocacy is written about in nursing ethics texts it often implies that it is the doctors who place patients in need of an advocate. This sets up a less than collegial situation between nursing and medicine and hardly provides a good starting point for teamwork.

The ethics literature in both nursing and medicine draws, then, on a variety of ethical theory and principles and puts discussion of cases and practice situations high on the agenda. The central theme of this book is that nursing and medical ethics might be better conceived of and played out as health care ethics. The reason for this is that the focus should be less on the professions and more on the patients and the nature of care, particularly the moral dimension of care. It is perhaps also the case that the interplay between the two perspectives on ethics, that of nursing and that of medicine, has been neglected, and the working out of a health care ethics will go some way to remedy this.

By taking a look at the day to day workings of health care and the social organisation of clinical practice we can gain an understanding of how the moral decisions are arrived at.

NOTES

1   The intensive care data come from an empirical study concerned with ethics in intensive care nursing. The data comprised transcripts from interviews with 24 experienced intensive care nurses. They were working in general adult intensive care, paediatric intensive care and cardiac surgery. Methodologically, the work followed a qualitative approach, drawing on the ideas of Glaser and Strauss (1967). The resultant analysis, whilst not generalisable in the quantitative sense, allows extrapolation of ideas.

2   The work of Jennings (1986; 1990) has influenced my approach to the study of intensive care ethics. These ideas were first published in a paper in *Social Science and Medicine* (Melia 2001).

3   Aristotle's *Nicomachean ethics*, so called as it was produced by Aristotle's son Nicomachus, is one of the most influential works in moral philosophy. The 1976 translation used in this book is by J.A.K. Thomson.

ii intensive care admission and withdrawal

THE PROPER USE OF INTENSIVE CARE

The literature concerned with the ethics of intensive care, or indeed with the nature of intensive care, returns constantly to a central theme, that of the proper use of the ICU. To know when to admit and when to stop treatment is the issue here, but it is rarely expressed in such terms. However when we examine what is said and written on the matter, it clearly comes down to the fact that intensive care is an expensive resource which for clinical, moral and fiscal reasons must be used appropriately (Audit Commission 1999; Vella et al. 2000). The central defining issue should be a clinical one, responding to the questions 'Does intensive care have anything to offer this patient?' and 'Will the patient benefit from this service?'

In this chapter this central question of the proper use of intensive care is addressed. I argued in the first chapter that the social context within which the ethical issues arise and are handled is important because the moral dimension of care cannot be divorced from the context within which it arises. Social considerations add to the already difficult situation because medical decisions involving intensive care admission are not straightforward. Medicine is not a precise science, and it is characterised by uncertainty (Atkinson 1984; 1995; Fox 1957; 1959; 1980; McIntosh 1977). Even if the clinical decisions could always be deemed to be clear-cut, leaving no room for debate, they still have to be effected in the world of social relationships and values. As it is, clinical decisions are often far from clear-cut when the possibility of admission to intensive care arises. And, even when the clinical view is that intensive care cannot help, or indeed would not be in the interests of the patient, the translation of that view into action is a complex social process involving clinicians and the patient and his or her significant others.[1] In fact, as we see from various studies in medical sociology, the arrival at the decision is also a social process involving negotiation (Anspach 1987; Chambliss 1996; Melia 2001; Seymour 2000; Strauss 1978; Strauss et al. 1985; Zussman 1992).

Intensive care now occupies a central place in health care and so the likelihood of the inappropriate use of intensive care could be said to have increased. This is not necessarily a criticism of physicians, more a comment on the state of twenty-first century health care. Seymour, in a study of death and dying in intensive care, sums up the situation when she says, 'Intensive care reflects the modern preoccupation with the mastery of disease and the eradication of untimely death' (2000: 103).

There are two critical points in the management of an intensive care patient: first when decisions have to be made about admission to the unit; and secondly if decisions have to be made about whether to withdraw treatment at some later stage when it is concluded that what is on offer in intensive care is not benefiting the patient. The decision to admit or not is essentially one about whether to withhold treatment or to go ahead and turn on the full works, as it were, in the ICU. It is the other side of the coin to a decision to withdraw, which may come later if the intensive care route turns out not to be in the patient's best interests.

Baldock says that:

In many ways intensive care flies in the face of the current philosophy of health care delivery. It provides expensive rescue care to a small number of people, of whom a substantial minority do not benefit, with minimal impact on the health of communities. (1995: 1612)

Baldock is setting the argument for intensive care in rather utilitarian terms, and if we were to follow that line of argument intensive care would not be so prominent or prevalent. Campbell (1984: 64) makes a similar point about a utilitarian argument leaving a good deal of need off the health care agenda: sick neonates, he says, would not be included in a utilitarian calculus. However, there are the more general principles of beneficence and non-maleficence, not to mention justice, which also drive society to want to provide for its vulnerable minorities.

This drive to do good has to be tempered with the caution to do no harm. The burdens and benefits offered by the ICU are a prime example of such a dilemma. The temptation is to see intensive care as a service which should be open to all in a 'let's give it a go' sense. Whilst the range of patients who may benefit from intensive care is wide, it should be reserved for those who are likely to benefit from it. Smith and Neilsen say that decisions should be 'based on the concept of potential benefit. Patients who are too well to benefit or those with no hope of recovering to an acceptable quality of life should not be admitted' (1999: 1544). Smith and Neilsen are right, but again uncertainty is an important factor here, as the idea of potential benefit requires an element of prediction and an idea of the prognosis. The difficulty lies in deciding who will benefit and who is more likely to raise the issue of withdrawal of treatment when it becomes clear that the ICU is merely serving to delay an inevitable death rather than providing the interim support needed for dysfunctional or failing organs to recover. The quality of life is an issue which exercises those engaged in debates in both medical and nursing ethics and increasingly the law is involved. We will examine this question in relation to persistent vegetative state (PVS) in Chapter 4.

Once a decision to admit has been taken, intensive care is a costly business. Bion in a *British Medical Journal* editorial noted one study (Sage et al. 1986) which showed that 'it costs twice as much to die in intensive care than it does to survive' (1995: 682). He goes on to say that 'in a recent British study [Atkinson et al. 1994] the 15% of 3,600 patients who died after admission to the intensive care unit consumed 38% of the unit's budget'.

The question of whether it is perhaps better not to admit in the first place than to run into the difficulty of withdrawal of treatment is a difficult but crucial one. The universal care instinct has an appeal: however, the difference between 'playing god' and exercising good professional judgement is never more acute than in the decision to treat aggressively or to let nature take its course. The point at which the decision to admit or to refuse admission to the ICU is taken is a critical one in relation to taking decisions about clinical need and resources. The question that hovers over the decision is whether it would have been better not to admit in the first place than to run into the difficulty of withdrawal.

In my study of ethics and intensive care, during a discussion of the complications of coronary bypass surgery, one senior ICU nurse said:

> R5: There is that sort of little window of time, you know, when somebody has had their operation, maybe they've had a perioperative event [something has gone wrong temporarily] or an event post-op, and there is just that little window where I don't know, physiologically if you can just say 'let's let that person die'. But, if you don't take that opportunity you then can't let somebody die because you'd be killing them. I am not sure if there is a real difference, but I feel that there is, I feel there is a little window there ... once you start you know the inotropes, or whatever, you then can't stop the ...
> KM: It is like Magnus Magnusson [quiz master], 'I've started so I'll finish.'[2]
> R5: Yes, that is exactly right and you know so you are at the end of the bed. You're seeing this patient, it is really dreadful and you don't know who it could happen to and unfortunately even when you CT scan them you can't tell very much – diffuse brain injury you just really don't know how that person is going to recover. And as the nurse at the end of the bed it is very, very hard to cope with and you have relatives sitting and they have no idea. You

know they just think 'oh the person will wake up and they will be fine' or, 'no they won't wake up at all', you know.

Seymour (2000) makes a similar point when she talks of the possibility of allowing a natural death in ICU. Running alongside what she refers to as the 'front stage' world of intensive care – by which she means that experienced by patients and their relatives – is, she says,

the behind the scenes activity whereby clinicians struggle to establish whether or not death is imminent and try to construct a case that justifies the withdrawal of 'active' medical treatment such that 'natural death' can occur. This is the vexed question of distinguishing between 'killing' and 'letting die'. (2000: 90)

On this same question moral philosophers argue as to whether there is a distinction to be made between withholding and withdrawing treatment. One line of argument is that if the good outcome lies in the peaceful death of the patient once the clinical judgement on prognosis is that it is futile to continue, then whether this is brought about by withholding the treatment in the first place, or by stopping it having started it, is of little moment. The outcome is the same. If we accept that in some cases the outcome of death is the right one and that this would be the likely eventuality after a burdensome time in ICU, it can be argued that not to admit in the first place would be a reasonable and morally sound action.

However, given the uncertainty which surrounds prognosis, such moral calculation is less easily effected in the clinical setting. There is also a strong emotional element to the question of how to act for the best, and so giving the benefit of the doubt will often lead to admission to ICU even when the strong likelihood is that the outcome will be poor and in fact the patient's experience may be the worse for having been given a 'chance' in the ICU. There is considerable debate about the efficacy of intensive care, some of it centring on the mortality after discharge from ICU (Daly et al. 2001). McPherson (2001) argues for the randomised control trial (RCT) in order to demonstrate efficacy; this too raises ethical issues. Also, according to Liddle et al. (1994) and Adrian et al. (1995), some over-optimistic expectations of cardio-pulmonary resuscitation are held by both health care staff and the public.

It is the liberal admission policy, despite the criteria for use of the ICU, which can lead to situations where the decision to withdraw is difficult. The Audit Commission note for example that the 'critical care units may become the backstop for a poorly performing hospital. Poor general care can result in patients needing critical care' (1999: 48).

Intensive care is now such a familiar part of the range of treatment options that to raise questions about its use is becoming increasingly difficult. Criteria for admission are theoretically reasonably well defined, but in practice the grey areas outstrip the black and white. Decisions to admit are often made in emergency and fraught circumstances, and once the patient is admitted the momentum of intensive care can take over. Decisions about continuing treatment are by and large medical decisions as they are part of the diagnosis and management of treatment responsibilities of medical staff. However, once the patient is in the ICU the prevailing organisational structure is that of the multidisciplinary team, and so nurses are far more likely to be involved.

All of this has to be considered in the light of the generally accepted criteria for admission to the ICU. Smith and Neilsen summarise these in terms of intensive care being appropriate for

> patients requiring or likely to require advanced respiratory support, patients requiring support of two or more organ systems, and patients with chronic impairment of one or more organ systems who require support for an acute reversible failure of another organ. (1999: 1544)

They also note that early referral is important, stating that 'If referral is delayed until the patient's life is clearly at risk, the chances of full recovery are jeopardised' (1999: 1544). Given this last caveat, it is not surprising that judgements tend to err on the side of caution when it comes to admission and not withholding intensive care. This necessarily tends to lead to difficult decisions about continuing or withdrawing treatment.

McHaffie and Fowlie (1996) sum up the problems surrounding the admission decision in a discussion of factors which influence decisions to withdraw treatment in neonatal intensive care. In a discussion of their interview data they describe the experiences and views of staff on the units in these terms:

> Prior to entering this speciality they had fairly strong ideas about what was right to do in terms of treatment but the experience had confused their certainty. They saw for themselves that babies could not be readily categorised and conceptualised. They were brought face to face with advances in technology and knowledge whilst at the same time confronting the limits of modern medicine. There were profound and diverse influences preventing the drawing of straight and hard lines. Not least among these influences was the fact that children defy predictions. It was very sobering to consider withdrawing treatment on a baby and perhaps years later to be brought face to face with that child enjoying a good quality of life. (1996: 79)

THE DECISION TO WITHDRAW TREATMENT

When we argue from one set of circumstances to another, in this case withdrawing treatment once started and withholding it in the first place, the caution is raised that it may lead to undesirable outcomes. The worry is that the analogy may be faulty and lead to poor conclusions: this is the slippery slope or 'wedge' (as in 'thin end of') argument. Beauchamp and Childress (1989) argue that we need to be clear about what is covered in these arguments. One form of the wedge argument focuses on the moral reasoning employed and the logical distinctions made between different actions. This means that if we argue for one course of action in one circumstance it may logically point to similar action in another situation – action which in the latter case we would generally consider to be wrong. Beauchamp and Childress (1989) cite as an example abortion, which if deemed to be right in one set of circumstances may logically imply a justification of infanticide in another. A similar argument is made in debates about gene manipulation and disability, where a desire to remove the possibility of a genetic condition, so the argument goes, implies that those living with that condition are somehow diminished by it. This line of argument rests on Kantian notions of universalisability, which would call for similar cases to be treated in a similar way. Taking up the abortion example, if a severely damaged foetus should be aborted, then a severely damaged baby should be killed. Beauchamp and Childress (1989) draw on Ramsey's (1978) work in which he argues that ethical and legal mistakes are repeated because of the universalisability argument. Ramsey says:

> it is quite clear that at the point of medical, legal and ethical intersections at the edges of life ... the so-called wedge argument is an excellent one. This is true because legal principles and precedents are systematically designed to apply to other cases as well. This is the way the law 'works' ... also the way moral reasoning 'works' from case to similar case. (1978: 306–7)

There are others who would claim a moral distinction between withholding and withdrawing, arguing that the latter is a less morally defensible action as it involves denial of something which was there.

Beauchamp and Childress (2001) discuss the distinctions made between withholding and withdrawing, the former being the situation where the treatment is never started and the latter when it is stopped. Beauchamp and Childress introduce the idea of withholding and withdrawing in terms of a discussion of the principle of non-maleficence, the harm being the forgoing of life-sustaining treatment, centring on omission or commission, i.e. withholding or eventually stopping. Even when withdrawal has been decided upon, differences of opinion exist with regard to what to withdraw: ventilation, but maintain hydration and other treatments; or stop all forms of treatment. Returning intravenous (IV) lines or naso-gastric tubes when they become dislodged is sometimes regarded as less problematic. Beauchamp and Childress say:

Some who had opposed stopping treatments felt comfortable about not inserting the IV line again because they viewed the action as withholding rather than withdrawing ... Others viewed the provision of artificial nutrition and hydration as a single process and felt that inserting the IV line again was simply restarting or continuing what had been interrupted. For them, not restarting was equivalent to withdrawing and thus (unlike withholding) morally wrong. (2001: 120)

Beauchamp and Childress link this reluctance on the part of caregivers to withdraw to the idea of a causal relationship between the withdrawal and death, whereas they say, 'they are not responsible if they never initiate a life-sustaining treatment'. Another source of discomfort with this, Beauchamp and Childress say, is that the caregivers somehow think that to withdraw treatment is to breach the expectations of the patient and to promise contractual obligations which don't exist if the treatment is simply withheld. Beauchamp and Childress conclude that whilst these various opinions are understandable, the distinction between withholding and withdrawing is 'both irrelevant and dangerous' (2001: 121). They say the distinction is in any case unclear, and even if it was clear, 'not starting and stopping can both be justified, depending on circumstances. Both not starting and stopping can cause a patient's death, and both can be instances of allowing to die. Both can even be instances of killing' (2001: 121).

The judgement on the rightness and wrongness of withholding and withdrawing is made upon the question of whether or not the doctor has an obligation not to withhold or withdraw. Beauchamp and Childress say that:

If a physician has a duty to treat then omission of treatment breaches the duty, whether withholding or withdrawing is involved: but if a physician does not have a duty to treat, or has a duty not to treat, then omission of either type involves no more violation. Indeed, if a physician has a duty not to treat, it would be a moral violation not to withdraw the treatment if it has already begun. (2000: 121)

This brings us back to the Hippocratic-based principle to do no harm and to a consideration of medical futility. Beauchamp and Childress conclude that it is the 'benefits and burdens of the treatment as judged by the patient or authorised surrogate that should be the main concern in determining how to act' (2001: 120).

A further point from Beauchamp and Childress is that 'Giving a priority to withholding over withdrawing also can lead to over-treatment in some cases – that is, to continue a treatment that is no longer beneficial or desirable for the patient' (2001: 122). Less obviously, they note too that it can lead to under-treatment. The worry of patients and families is that they will be unable to escape treatment once it starts, and 'To circumvent this problem they become reluctant to authorize the technology, even when it could be beneficial' (2001: 122). Beauchamp and Childress also say that health care professionals often come 'to show the same reluctance'. This was mentioned in the interview extract earlier in this chapter, where an ICU staff nurse spoke of the 'window of time' in which to call a halt.

Seymour (2000) has some useful comments on this matter. In her work she is concerned with the ways in which the withdrawal of treatment is managed in intensive care. The central idea is that the accomplishment of a 'natural death' in the intensive care setting is a matter of negotiation and should be regarded as a social process. Seymour's book is about how the decision to remove life support is managed when it turns out not to have been in the patient's interests. The study is therefore concerned with clinical decisions and how these are arrived at and the ethical, social and financial implications of these decisions.

Seymour's point is that medical decision making at the bedside is an interactional accomplishment involving negotiation and renegotiation of the technical data, the trajectory of the known technical dying and how this is aligned with the seen and felt bodily dying. In other words Seymour is saying that the physiological measurements and data which indicate that the body is failing are relied upon as the hard evidence that the patient is actually dying. She draws on Atkinson's (1995) work and examines the pace of the death indicated by clinical data (test results etc.) which is available to clinicians. Seymour is interested in the 'way in which medical staff assemble and "read" clinical data from a complex range of sources' (2000: 33). She explores the way in which in intensive care it is the 'shared meaning of that data that is negotiated in terms that define patients as either "dying" or "recoverable", and how a framework is developed to guide and delimit future medical action' (2000: 33). The main concern is to ensure that the withdrawal of treatment is the best decision to take, and that it is taken on sound technical grounds. Because of the recognised reluctance that goes with this course of action, the moral issues are more readily handled if the death can be seen to be inevitable and not as a direct consequence of withdrawal.

Beauchamp and Childress make the point that professionals and family members alike often feel more comfortable withholding than they do withdrawing. They say:

> They sense that the decisions to stop treatments are more momentous and consequential than decisions not to start them. Stopping a respirator, for example, seems to cause a person's death, whereas not starting the respirator does not seem to have this direct causal role. (2001: 120)

This is the opposite of the 'well at least we tried' position, where the argument is that there is less difficulty in withdrawing because at least the opportunity was offered. Neither approach can be said to be without emotional overtones: this is the reality of intensive care. A decision is the point at which an understanding of how these actions are played out, how they feel in practice, is essential, and it is important to consider not simply the philosophical arguments for favouring one line of action over another. In other words it is the point at which moral philosophy and a sociological analysis of the clinical situation can usefully be brought together.

MEDICAL FUTILITY

Medical futility is a relevant concept here as it denotes the point at which to withdraw is the right thing to do. If prediction of outcomes were more precise it could also be useful in making the 'when not to start' decision, that is when to withhold. Aside from the uncertainty it is arguable that the general professional drive to do something, the Hippocratic impera-tive to help, causes those making the decision to admit the patient to the ICU, when it would have been a better idea not to admit, that is to with-hold treatment. This puts admitting into the stronger position, which then makes the question of withdrawal an issue. By this I mean that there is a tendency to over-admit because we cannot predict well enough what the outcome of the decision will be. The culture then encourages the continuation of effort and a reluctance to give up once started.

So whilst moral philosophers can argue as to whether there is or is not a difference between withholding and withdrawing, the feeling on the ground is that withdrawing is, as Beauchamp and Childress (2001) have it, more consequential than withholding. Sometimes decisions to withhold treatment, or failing to admit, are made because of shortages of intensive care beds. As Bennett and Bion put it, 'under-resourced hospi-tals may have to refuse admission to those who otherwise would be admitted' (1999: 1468–9). This situation can be said to be much more a case of withholding, when that term has a negative connotation. It is not due to any fault in the clinical team, but because of resources and wider political questions of health care funding. Withholding for good clinical, and thereby ethical, reasons when it is judged that admission will be of no benefit, and indeed may be to the detriment of the patient's wellbe-ing, should perhaps be seen as a good and positive action, even though on the face of it to withhold seems to be a negative thing to do.

All of which brings us back to the question of medical futility. This is well summed up by Winter and Cohen:

> withdrawal of treatment is an issue in intensive care medicine because it is now possible to maintain life for long periods with-out any hope of recovery. Intensive care is usually a process of

supporting organ systems, but it does not necessarily offer a cure.
(1999: 306)

They go on to say that 'Prolonging the process of dying is not in the
patient's interests as it goes against ethical principles of beneficence and
non-maleficence' (1999: 306). These authors also point out that about
70% of deaths in ICUs occur after withdrawal of treatment, and note that
'This is not euthanasia. The cause of death remains the underlying disease process, and treatment is withdrawn as it has become futile.' The
point they make about this being nothing to do with euthanasia is
important: intensive care is about organ failure, most often multiple
organ failure, and therefore euthanasia is not an issue in this sphere of
medicine.

The high incidence of death after withdrawal of treatment is a function of the tendency to err on the side of caution and to admit to the ICU
if there is any possibility of recovery, even if this is not very likely. In
other words, many of those admitted to the ICU probably never stood a
chance. Again, we are looking at the two sides of the same coin: to admit
is to decide not to withhold; if that decision turns out to be a poor one,
then withdrawal is likely to ensue. It is more a matter of timing, a matter of the ICU delaying the inevitable. Zussman makes this clear when
he says that 'the ICU staff live in a moral universe of limited liability,
what happens afterwards is not their responsibility' (1992: 43). This is
perhaps a rather harsh statement, but it contains more than an element
of truth.

At the heart of the debate about whether there is a moral difference
between withholding and withdrawing treatment should be this question of futility and a focus on the principles of beneficence and non-
maleficence. The problem is that medical futility is in itself a contested
matter. A comment from an American professor of law and medicine is
interesting on this matter: 'Many aspects of modern medicine provoke
spirited ethical argument, but few engender as much disagreement
about what exactly is at issue as does the futility debate' (Capron 1997:
ix).

He goes on to make a point similar to that made by Zussman (1992)
about the shift in power in these matters of life and death. There has
been a shift from the medical profession to the law and the patient via
the developments in the recognition of patient autonomy and informed
consent. In other words the professional dominance of medicine has
been nudged aside by the legal notions of autonomy and informed consent. Capron says:

As characterised by some, physicians have become pathetic char-
acters in a modern day Molière play, technically sophisticated servants doing the bidding of their patients. Professionals with this
perception feel misused and justify their rebelliousness by invok-

> ing medical futility. The simple recognition of the limits of medi-
> cine's power to cure and to extend life denotes that health care
> professionals should not be obliged to provide further treatment
> or, more powerfully, that they would exceed their role-based
> authority as healers to continue to do so. Yet other commentators
> claim that medical futility is an empty concept that does not pro-
> vide any ground for decision that would not be present had the
> concept never been coined. They characterise medical futility as
> nothing more than a cover for physicians' rearguard action to
> regain the dominance in decision making that they possessed
> before autonomy and informed consent shifted authority to
> patients and their families in the 1960s. (1997: ix)

In a paper in the collection introduced by Capron, Brody (1997) argues
the case for the utility of the concept of medical futility. Brody says that
arguments which seem difficult in the abstract often become more
tractable at a practical, policy level. Thus, he says,

> it may be at the practical level – particularly by asking what sorts
> of discussions we want to take place within health care institu-
> tions – that we will eventually come to understand what futility
> means and what its appropriate limitations are. (1997: 1)

This is another example of bringing moral philosophy and sociological
analysis together.

In summary, once the decision to admit has been made – that is, not
to withhold – the possible outcomes are either a success, that is recovery,
or a need to withdraw treatment at some later point. It can be argued
that if the better action is to let nature take its course and not to treat
aggressively, then whether this comes about early on by withholding or
later by withdrawing is of little moment as the upshot is the same. We
have seen then that it is the social context, the emotional aspect, that
makes withdrawing intrinsically more difficult than withholding. This
may be because we don't really address withholding too closely; there is
more of a tendency to admit to the ICU if we can.

An Audit Commission survey showed that of '103 units that col-
lected information on organ failure, on average 12% of patients in ICUs
had three or more organs in failure. Also, 25% of units had 20% of such
patients' (1999: 42). One clinician in the survey interviews said that 'most
patients admitted with three or more organs in failure die'. His view was
that 'a unit that admits high numbers of such patients is misusing
resources and should allow such patients to die, without further intervention, in a more suitable environment' (1999: 42).

The emotional difficulty experienced in withdrawing is mediated
by questions of justice and fairness which tend to make withholding a
difficult decision to take. This coupled with the inherent uncertainty of
critical illness, noted earlier, makes it much more likely that admission

to the ICU will take place if there is capacity and staff to allow this. On a more general level, whilst intensive care is a speciality, its existence has knock-on effects for other areas of health care. Elective surgery lists may be cancelled if intensive care beds are used for post-operative difficulties and other emergencies.

There is a problem with trying to run a complex emergency service alongside a planned service. On average around 25% of admissions are planned, for elective surgery. The rest are the result of emergencies (Audit Commission 1999: 15). This is compounded by the fact that intensivists are usually anaesthetists on a duty rota for theatre. This wider remit is a consequence of the small scale of UK intensive care compared with units in other parts of Europe and in the United States. This small scale makes the balancing of emergency admissions and the planned admission of complicated post-operative patients difficult. This constant juggling of resources in order to facilitate admissions is a factor, albeit an unwelcome one, in decisions about admission and discharge (Lapsley and Melia 2001).

When the argument about whether to invoke intensive care for a patient focuses upon withholding and withdrawal debates, it detracts from the more central question of 'Is intensive care appropriate here?' This brings us back again to the notion of medical futility. Brody (1997) says that there are two questions involved. The first is whether there are medical interventions about which we can be sufficiently confident in terms of their outcome as to label them 'futile'. And secondly, if this is possible, he asks: 'Are physicians entitled, or indeed obligated, to refuse to provide those interventions to the patient in question, even if the treatment is requested or demanded by the patient or appropriate surrogate?' (1997: 1).

Brody says that those who argue that the notion of medical futility is unhelpful, or even a dangerous concept, do so on the grounds that these questions are too hard to answer. He points to a tendency to rely on the physiological outcomes and to test the futility question against the outcomes in terms of organs rather than people. He cites cardio-pulmonary resuscitation (CPR) as a development in medical care which has proved to be beneficial to a very small number of patients, and says:

> the success of CPR led to a phenomenon fairly typical of modern medicine – the uncritical use of technology that has proved beneficial for a small number of patients for treating other patients who have not been shown to benefit. CPR soon became the standard reaction to any patient in any US health care setting who suffered a cardiac arrest. (1997: 4)

Brody notes that experience and research have shown that CPR has a good success rate in the population of patients for whom it was originally designed, coronary care patients. The label 'futile' is appropriate in many other cases: this led to the introduction of the 'do not resuscitate' (DNR) or 'not for resuscitation' (NFR) order. This moves the problem on a little, but the central question of medical uncertainty remains. And, as with the withhold or withdrawal argument, the tendency will be to err on the side of caution, or more accurately of action. This often manifests itself as a reluctance in doctors to write NFR orders; their reluctance is matched by an eagerness on the part of nurses to have some clarity on the matter and to know what an individual patient's resuscitation status is.

The 'not for resuscitation' order is a very difficult area for the two professional groups. Doctors are reluctant to put the order in writing; nurses like to know where they stand. Both positions are understandable, but not compatible. The consultant, taking account of the views of colleagues and the patient (if this is possible) and relatives, is responsible for the decision. Nurses may then be put in the position of acting where they think that they should not or, conversely, not acting where they think that they should. As we have seen with the debates about withholding and withdrawing, it is very difficult to stop once a course of action has been started upon. It is not possible to turn society's expectations in another direction once they are set on new possibilities: reproductive medicine is a case in point. The medical profession has invested considerable effort in trying to get the legal and moral balance right in the withholding and withdrawing of life-prolonging treatment. The advice in a professional publication (British Medical Association 1999; 2001) takes account of the multidisciplinary nature of health care work. It also makes it clear that whilst the decision is, at law, a medical one, the views of other members of the team, and the patient (where possible) or the relatives, should be sought. The social context is also recognised, evidenced by this passage in the introduction:

> Matters of life and death give rise to emotive and impassioned debate. Such responses cannot and should not be ignored. The symbolic importance of appearing to 'give up' on some patients cannot be over-estimated and sensitivity is required to ensure that such impressions are not given. As we stress throughout, good communications, listening to all relevant parties and thoroughly investigating the options are central to good decision making. The decisions addressed in this document may generate conflicting views. This guidance urges a cautious and thoughtful approach to such decisions, recognising the difficult areas of ethical tension and legal uncertainties and the possibility of divergence of medical opinion, whilst attempting to provide practical assistance to those patients and health professionals who must confront these issues. (1999: xviii)

There have been cases in the press where patients have found NFR marked on their notes and they have been unaware of this fact and no discussion has taken place. Also some hospital policies have led to what might be seen to be an over-the-top openness on the matter whereby any patient in the hospital has the question of resuscitation discussed with them. This policy includes cases where there is no likelihood of an arrest or, if it were to happen, the resuscitation would be of no avail and so the discussion served no goal of beneficence with the patient or the family. It is argued by the doctors involved that such discussions with patients cause more upset than is warranted; the principle of non-maleficence is breached. This is an example of one more principle, respect for autonomy, being followed, but when we examine how it plays out on a daily basis the outcome is not always in the patient's best interest. In fact it can be said to be doing more harm than good. Brody uses the cardio-pulmonary resuscitation (CPR) example to point up the flaw in the anti-futility argument. His reasoning is that if those who wish to deny medical futility have it that doctors should not make unilateral decisions (clinical judgement) about whether or not to start CPR, they should be equally in favour of patient or family consent being involved in stopping the CPR. Brody makes the point clearly thus:

> No-one on the anti-futility side of the debate, however, seems upset that physicians are allowed to make reasonable judgements about what is working and not working and unilaterally decide to stop the code [resuscitation] based on those judgements. The reason it does not bother them and does not bother the majority of patients and families is obvious: when one considers all aspects of the practical situation, no other policy makes sense. This feature of how CPR decisions are made in the real world illustrates conclusively to me that those on the anti-futility side of the debate are caught in a logical contradiction. If they are so worried about unilateral physician decision making whether to start CPR, they should be equally worried about unilateral physician decision making about when to stop CPR. (1997: 5–6)

Brody's conclusion is that the concept of medical futility is difficult because we try to discuss it in terms of autonomy or justice and so 'demand abstract terms but precise definitions'. This he says will simply leave the issue muddled. The arguments about futile care are used when a patient or their proxy wants to refuse treatment.

Zussman (1992) argues that whilst medicine is constrained by the law as to what treatments can and cannot be withdrawn, physicians retain their right to determine what constitutes aggressive treatment and non-aggressive treatment and so reclaim their clinical discretion. Zussman sums it up like this:

> Physicians avoid beginning those treatments they believe the law proscribes them from withdrawing. By assimilating the distinction between those treatments they cannot withdraw and those they

> can into a more general distinction between more and less
> aggressive treatment, they justify their avoidance in terms of the
> patient's best interest. But unlike a distinction between more and
> less aggressive treatment based on degrees of invasiveness or
> risk of treatments, a distinction based on the ability to withdraw
> treatment does not speak so clearly to the patient's best interest
> as to the physician's freedom of action. Thus, while the prohibi-
> tions on withdrawing treatment limit the physician's discretion,
> their use of the concept of 'aggressive' treatment helps restore it.
> (1992: 137–8)

Zussman's point is similar to other comments on the uncertainty surrounding diagnosis and the inevitable variation in clinical judgements
which follows. We can see from the various analyses of clinicians at
work in ICUs that the process of coming to a decision is a social one
focusing on technical data, framed by law but inevitably including a
moral judgement. Zussman puts this eloquently when he says of the difference in practice in relation to withdrawal of treatment in the ICUs in
the two hospitals he studied:

> Thus, buried in technical discussions are deep and largely unar-
> ticulated differences in general orientations ... In this difference –
> masked by the language of prognosis and diagnosis, by the
> results of laboratory tests and probability estimates – is the open
> moral space of American medicine. It is a space quickly filled with
> physicians' values. (1992: 133)

Since the Quinlan case[3] in the USA established the right to terminate
treatment, the question of withdrawing the treatment has been on the
agenda. The courts are involved[4] but the principle is now generally
accepted that there is no need to continue with futile treatment when it
can bring no good outcome. More problematic is the situation where the
patient or family request treatment which is considered by the medical
staff to be futile.

PROFESSIONAL RESPONSIBILITY AND
THE WITHDRAWAL OF TREATMENT

The decision to treat or not is one of the defining points in distinguishing between nursing and medical responsibilities. Nurses are less
involved in the decision to admit to ICU than they are in decisions about
withdrawal of treatment once the patient is in the unit (Melia 2001). It is,
then, often the case that nurses feel that they are left in the position of
following through on decisions which were taken by the doctors. As we
have already noted, issues and circumstances beyond the ICU can influence the admission decision. The fact that for much of the time nurses
are acting on the decisions of medicine is usually presented as a prob-

lem. Nurses often claim to have a better knowledge of the patient by virtue of the long periods of time spent with them. On the other hand it is the medical consultant who carries the legal responsibility for the management of the case and thus for any decision to withdraw treatment. The doctor's intermittent relationship with the patient is usually portrayed in nursing ethics texts as one from which less knowledge of the patient is developed; when decisions about limiting or withdrawing treatment are being taken, nurses emphasise their close relationship with the patients and relatives, and so a moral agenda is emphasised.

Nurses will argue that they have a more detailed knowledge of the patient by virtue of prolonged proximity. This is where the case for the nurse as the patient's advocate comes from. The idea behind this advocacy argument is that by virtue of their position *vis-à-vis* the patient and relatives they are best placed to know what would be in the patient's best interests. Zussman (1992) argues that the fact that nurses in intensive care have responsibility for care, and less for cure, does not make them 'angels', nor does it provide a basis for the advocacy role. He says that it is their technical skills that ICU nurses are recognised for and it is those skills which earn them the respect of their medical colleagues:

> It is technical skill, not empathy or a special faculty for kindness, that is recognised and rewarded by physicians and the hospital hierarchy. Nurses may concern themselves with care rather than cure, with the social and emotional aspects of illness rather than physiology, but in the ICU they are rarely able to express that concern ... They are not patients' advocates. They are not 'angels of mercy'. Like physicians, they have become technicians. (1992: 80)

Nursing and medicine have different and interdependent roles within the health care team. Nurses have less input into the decision to admit to the ICU and so the starting point for the withdrawal discussion is different for nurses and doctors. The admission decision is one based on diagnosis and the prospects for managing the case through to a good outcome. This is the province of medicine.

In my study, a senior ICU nurse reflected on the vexed question of whether a patient should have been admitted to ICU in the first place:

> *KM*: What is the nursing view on that? Do you get involved in the decision to admit?
> *HC*: Well, you see unfortunately, Kath, you don't, what will happen is say like now I went back and they wanted to admit somebody, it should normally be a specialist registrar, consultant decision, so obviously, you won't take a phone call from an SHO on a medical ward and the patient's coming. So you have probably got somebody quite senior ... will phone up the unit and give the details and what I will do at that point is, just as if they were saying to me, I know it is hard to put an age, but say 88-year-old lady

> X, Y and Z and I will sort of say things like 'Well what was her qual-
> ity of life like before this?' I will ask appropriate questions which
> you know that the anaesthetist would have asked but you just
> want to make it clear in your head that this has all been through.
> And if it was a case where you thought, hang on a minute, this just
> doesn't seem to be an intensive care patient, or a kind of border-
> line intensive care, I would express that view, but at the end of the
> day that decision is going to be made by the consultant anaes-
> thetist. You know they make the final decisions but what you can
> do is just express your opinions, concerns etc. and then they are
> admitted to the ICU.

The interview data from the ICU nurses suggest that nurses are very
much involved in the decisions about patient management once the
patient is in the ICU, even though there are often differences of opinion.
The impression which Chambliss (1996) conveys is somewhat different.
In rather vivid terms he says:

> the nurses will claim that physicians who persist with aggressive
> treatment are not truly caring for the patient (a basic function of
> nursing) and that this is immoral, simply wrong, morally wrong.
> Physicians will respond that the doctor's duty is to save the
> patient's life ... So nurses and doctors approach the patient with
> significantly different goals, and these are described in moral
> terms. (1996: 95–6)

Chambliss goes further and says that when there is a difference of opinion between medicine and nursing, nurses resort to the moral agenda:

> caring is also an ideological term, an idealised way of talking
> about nursing. It is openly used as a weapon in nurses' conflicts
> with physicians, to distinguish what nurses do (care) from what
> doctors do (cure), and to assert the nurses' moral superiority.
> (1996: 68)

The main point that Chambliss makes is that the position of nursing
within the hierarchy of professional workers in the hospital organisation
is that of subordinates to medicine. He argues therefore that they have
the problems that any occupational group working in an organisation
has with those in more superior positions. Chambliss has it that nurses
are often resorting to the moral arguments when they have no other
grounds upon which to win a debate. He goes so far as to say, and it has
to be conceded that he has something of a point, that

> much of the nursing literature suffers from an exaggerated ideal-
> ism, and many nurses will in effect say, 'I would do things differ-
> ently if I were in charge.' But they aren't in charge, and if they
> were, experience shows us that they would probably do things

the way people in charge do. (1996: 88)

Chambliss provides a sociological analysis of nursing ethics, and presents what he calls the 'social organisation of ethics'. On this view, nursing ethics is often more a manifestation of the power struggles between the two occupational groups, with nursing, the less powerful, resorting to moral argument as a means of achieving some control in a situation where medicine is the more powerful profession.

The position is arguably more subtle and complex than Chambliss allows. It may be that the ICU teams that I encountered (Melia 2001) were exceptionally collegial, although I have no reason to suppose that to have been the case. Seymour (2000) sheds some light on how the team works in the ICU. She argues that whilst medicine and nursing perceive their work differently in the ICU, nursing by co-operating with and recognising the 'medical interpretation of the patient prevents any breakdown in good, co-ordinated team effort'. As she puts it, this is

in spite of a comparatively high degree of autonomy and the 'total care' orientation of the nurses which compels them to reproduce the patient as a 'known', rather than a depersonalised entity. The co-operation of the nursing staff and their attention to the medically framed aspects of their role effectively subvert conflict between the professions. (2000: 65)

The less hierarchical analysis offered by Seymour is perhaps more of a contemporary reflection of the state of professional relationships in the ICU.

Walby et al. (1994: 85) undertook a study of medicine and nursing as 'professions in a changing health service', drawing mainly on interview data. Their purpose was to 'map the patterns of conflict and co-operation between doctors and nurses in a wide range of contexts'. With regard to ICUs they describe the respect of medicine and nursing for each other's work. In general they say that there is a tendency for doctors to delegate to other health workers 'tasks which have become simple or onerous'. They note that the practice of delegation ensures that the control of the work remains with medicine. This is not of course a new thought: Everett Hughes (1951) spoke of nurses delegating tasks to 'aides and maids', whilst at the same time taking on medical tasks. However, Walby et al. (1994) note that support was exhibited by medicine for the extending role of the nurse whereby nurses take on more responsibility. Walby et al. take this as a positive sign, saying 'this is not the response of a defensive profession under threat from a neighbouring professional rival' (1994: 85). Interestingly they note with some rather dated language, 'If doctors were to be threatened by the rising skill level of nurses, then ICU departments should have contained leading examples of this. In fact consultants were proud of the skill of their [sic] nurses and full of praise for their professionalism and ability.' With some irony, at least I hope so, they state that 'Somehow these skills were not perceived to stray onto any territory that the doctors wished to keep for themselves' (1994: 86).

These comments say a good deal about the relationship between the professions of medicine and nursing in the ICU. Some would argue that the position described leaves much to be desired, but at least there is teamworking of a sort and an absence of hostility. Those making a distinction between medical and nursing ethics, and I have been there (Melia 1989), argue that the difference lies in the way the issues present to the different professional groups and the practical problems they bring with them. So whilst many of the ethical issues that come up in health care present problems for medicine and nursing, the argument goes that it is the reaction to these issues that is profession specific and hence led medical and nursing ethics to develop in parallel, as separate but related entities. The footprints of this argument still inhabit my thinking, but on balance, as I argue in this book, I think that these perspectives are best pooled in an effort to understand health care ethics. The moves towards multidisciplinary practice, teamwork, blurring of professional boundaries and shared learning in a patient-led health service would support this view.

MEDICAL AND NURSING PERSPECTIVES ON WITHDRAWAL

The discussion here is based on work concerned with decisions to withdraw treatment in intensive care (Melia 2001). In situations of withdrawal the difference of opinion between nursing and medical staff was not so much a disagreement over the ethical issues, but more a function of the different roles and responsibilities within the health care team. Everyone understood the need for the decision to be taken carefully and that it was sometimes of necessity a lengthy business. Nonetheless, those in closest proximity to the patient, those who witnessed the reactions of the family and friends, tended to become impatient with consultants and the time they took to reach a decision. The senior nurses, by the same token of proximity, but this time to the consultants' viewpoint, tended to be the most understanding of the consultants' position. Some would go so far as to say that if the nurses had to take responsibility for the decision, rather than providing ethical commentary on it, it might be a different story – an echo of the position Chambliss (1996) takes. It has to be said that in these interviews the nurses who were working mostly at the bedside expressed sympathy for the consultants' position, but also admitted to being somewhat intolerant of it in practice. This type of comment was always made in the context of an understanding of the unevenness in the team when it comes to responsibility for clinical decisions. In my study, one very experienced intensive care nurse summed up the situation like this:

> if you were placed in that actual position ... you know, could I go home and sleep at night, thinking today I withdrew therapy, even if you knew within yourself it was the right thing to do, would I sleep soundly tonight knowing that?

It was clear that there is one ethical issue which is paramount in intensive care: it was mentioned, sooner or later (mostly sooner), by all the respondents. This was the question of coming to the decision to withdraw treatment from an intensive care patient. The complex nature of these withdrawal decisions is conveyed in the following extracts; both are from senior nurses in charge of the ICU.

> I think for me in intensive care it is very much the continuation of treatment and the withdrawal of treatment. And I think that what I feel gives you ethical dilemmas is when you sort of feel that we are carrying on and shouldn't be carrying on. And even though you are working very closely as a multidisciplinary team and you are obviously discussing it on a daily basis I sort of get the feeling that often it's the nursing staff who will reach the conclusion quicker than medical staff that enough is enough. Probably because you are with the patient say for about 12 hours and you are with the family and you just get sort of probably, just a better feel if you like, but I appreciate from the medical side they have obviously got to do, you know legally as well as everything else all their bits and pieces before they can reach the decision. It is not that there is kind of, you know nurses are right and the doctors are wrong, but I just think the actual time span can feel very sort of prolonged, particularly from a nursing point of view.

> I think the main one has to be this continuation of treatment and how active, probably yes the continuation of treatment but also the admission to ICU, I would say were the two things that caused, and continue I think to cause, nurses grief if you like. Not just because of the ethical issues but because of the differences between consultants.

Both of these extracts get straight to the central ethical question for intensive care nurses, namely the withdrawal of treatment. The interview data and sociological analyses bring out not only the fact of the decision but the way in which it plays out in the social context of practice. The nurses describe how the decision to withdraw is difficult, and whilst the decision itself is not always in dispute, it is the way in which it comes about that causes problems for the nursing staff. In fact many times during these interviews it became clear that nurses understand very well that the decision to withdraw takes time to arrive at, and that the consultant in charge of the ICU carries the legal responsibility for the decision and has to be satisfied that the decision is the right one. As we have noted, intensive care is a particularly difficult area in which to predict outcomes and this leads to periods of time in which the consultant is making sure that all avenues have been properly explored – periods of time which are difficult to get through for those closest to the minute by minute care of the patient. Typically those closest are the nurses at the bedside. However the junior doctors also spend a lot of time on the intensive care units and experience the same impatience and desire for decisions to be made promptly.

The following extract from the interview with the senior nurse in charge of the ICU serves to illustrate several issues which are examined in the remainder of this chapter (Melia 2001). She is discussing the medical management of the ICU, the fact that a group of anaesthetists rather than intensivists (these are usually anaesthetists who work solely within the ICU) work on a weekly rota on the ICU. This makes for some continuity and aids decision making, but it presents too the potential for problems at the handover from one consultant anaesthetist to another. The smooth running of an ICU, especially in the context of difficult decisions about withholding and withdrawing, depends upon close and good working relations between nursing and medicine.

> *HC:* What a lot of ICUs have done is where they used to have a different consultant on in charge every day, they now do it on a week basis, a week by week basis, because what would happen in the past is, this is no exaggeration, one day one consultant will be coming on saying 'right, if no improvement by tomorrow morning, withdrawing', and the other consultant comes on and goes like back to square one and starts all this aggressive care and 'why haven't we done X, Y and Z?' And literally changing the goalposts, you know markedly, each day. So I think having the same consultant on helps because you have got them there for a week, they are building up a picture, they are meeting the family and I think because you do liaise very closely with the doctors, I don't think you have any, I don't think now there is any kind of, not recently I have not come across any real sort of major issues, it is just more, that it does seem to go on longer sometimes for the nursing staff than it does the medical staff. As I said at the beginning, not because they are dragging their heels, or they just won't, but it is just ...

This senior nurse's comments are wide ranging but she is focusing yet again on the questions surrounding withholding and withdrawing treatment in intensive care. She notes that the period of coming to a decision is experienced by nurses as a more protracted business than it is for the doctors, largely because it is not the nurses' decision, yet they are closest to its consequences. She goes on to say that the 'drawn out' nature of decision making is a problem too for junior doctors. Later in the interview she describes very graphically a situation (not a rare event on the evidence of the rest of the data) of a patient being admitted where, with hindsight, it could be said that intensive care was not an appropriate choice of treatment. In describing the situation she demonstrates a sympathy with the medical perspective on the same situation.

> But I think what is really hard for the medical staff is very often, take for example we have got a patient on at the moment who came down from the medical ward last night, the anaesthetist was called up and he had the patient down within minutes and the patient was almost ready to collapse on the ward, now as it turns out now that they have got time to look back at the patient and the past medical history etc. this particular patient I think can do very little and be breathless in a chair at home and it was lung problems that she came down with. Now, I am not saying it is a right or wrong decision to bring the patient down, but I think very often for the anaesthetist called to wards, the patient is blue, about to arrest and you know you can't really start to kind of ethically debate, it is very much like this patient is going to die if we don't. Let's intubate them, get them to ICU and then you can sort of, you end up kind of stepping back. Now probably there are sometimes at that point the anaesthetists themselves think oh, dear, probably not the best of decisions. But I think it is the best decision with the information they are given at the time and the situation.

This senior intensive care nurse is describing the two sides of the coin which represent the main dilemma in intensive care: the withholding or withdrawing of treatment. In the cool light of moral philosophical debate the decisions seem clear, whereas in the messy world of clinical practice, the social context for the playing out of moral decisions, things are less clear-cut. The extract clearly demonstrates the nurse's understanding of the difficulties faced by the doctor who has to make the clinical decisions. It was often the case that nurses in describing their frustrations around the 'withdrawal' issue – frustrations shared by junior doctors – acknowledged, as does this nurse, the difficult decision that the consultant anaesthetist ultimately has to make. This acknowledgement can be seen as evidence of the importance of teamwork and the associated tendency to look for consensus in intensive care.

The situation can be summed up in a slight caricature of the two professions involved as a situation where medicine, concentrating as it does on prognosis, understandably takes time to withdraw. Nursing, on the other hand, takes a whole person view and so wants to move to a decision sooner.

In an interview-based study of ethics in ICUs there was a view expressed by the nurses who had experience of general intensive care, and of units where major cardiac surgery was undertaken, that the consultant anaesthetists tended to take a more all-round approach to the decision to withdraw compared with the surgeons involved (Melia 2001). Whilst it is generally the case that ICUs are anaesthetist-led, there were occasions described where the surgeons' views were at odds with more general intensive care opinion. It is perhaps not surprising to note that the nurses, whilst understanding the surgeons' viewpoint, tended to take the same line as the anaesthetists. The nurses I interviewed had more than 10 years of experience of intensive care and were used to the workings of the ICU team. They were therefore well placed to comment on the consequences for nursing practice in intensive care of there being times when the team was less than functional. These nurses with cardiac surgical unit experience described situations which posed perhaps most sharply the problem of long drawn out situations which led up to the withdrawal of treatment, as in the following extract from a senior nurse.

> In the general ICU the anaesthetist may say, 'this is hopeless', and will stop. In the cardiac surgery unit we very rarely let people die, we keep going on and on and on until they are no longer viable.

Seymour (2000) also shows how the nursing and medical perspectives in ICUs differ. This short extract from her fieldnotes illustrates the point well:

> [The senior registrar] sits next to me [Seymour] at the nurses' station and I ask him how he thinks Mrs Hall is: 'Mrs Hall? – oh she's OK. Well, let's put it like this, she's better than she was on Wednesday night, and I think she'll be OK eventually.' The G grade (senior) sister who is also sitting at the station gazes at him in almost a derisive manner and explodes. 'Ha!' The senior registrar responds to this expletive lamely: 'Oh well, maybe not, X doesn't agree with me.' Sister: 'She's got so many things wrong with her.' Senior registrar: 'That's true, but at least she's shown that she can put up her cardiac output to 6 litres from 4 yesterday – I know she is on noradrenaline but that is better.' (2000: 62)

Seymour's comment in her analysis is: 'The implication is that the nurse sees her role as primarily one of promoting Mrs Hall's comfort, rather than one of colluding in what may be a futile attempt to wean her from ventilation' (2000: 62).

An even more extreme example of this 'doing medicine' or even 'doing science' approach to intensive care comes in Zussman's (1992) work. One resident (junior medical staff) said:

> you don't have to look at the patient here, basically you don't have to really examine a patient ... Someone has a PA (pulmonary artery) line in, you don't have to listen to their lungs ... In that respect, with technology you don't have to deal with a patient,

examine a patient. The numbers, I feel, they are more reliable. (1992: 33)

And, as another put it, in a striking image in which the irrelevance of the patient's personhood becomes altogether apparent, 'In a way it's almost like veterinary medicine' (1992: 33).

This is clearly a rather extreme rendering of the situation in the ICU, and many physicians, and possibly vets, would not go along with it. It does, however very clearly draw out the point that Atkinson (1995) makes about 'reading the body'. As Atkinson puts it:

The body is sampled, invaded, measured and inspected, in order to yield images and information. Those data can then be scrutinised and interrogated elsewhere in the specialised departments and laboratories of the modern hospital ... It is in this way that the body is rendered legible. (1995: 61)

Atkinson goes on to show how the various specialists produce the care by talking and putting forward their interpretations of the data in order to render an accurate clinical picture. Atkinson says that 'a great deal of medical work and instruction was conducted in spoken performances. One could think of medical work in terms of rhetorical skills' (1995: 4). If this can be said of the process of arriving at the 'clinical picture', how much more powerful the idea is when we include the moral element.

The decision to withdraw is often carried out in stages: typically the nurses described this as 'leaving it 24 hours or 48 and then see'. During this time those by the bed space, nurses and junior medical staff, begin to perceive the futility of continuing treatment and start to push for a halt to be called sooner than those taking the decision would like. The consultant anaesthetists are responsible for the decision. The more long-standing experienced nursing staff tend to hold similar views. The latter, whether by dint of experience or less proximity to the hands-on care, take a view closer to that of the consultants who hold legal responsibility for management of the case (Melia 2001). These senior nurses witnessed both sides of the 'wait and see' experience and tended to lead, or at least prompt, the move towards withdrawal. In other words, they accepted the 24 hour wait but were quick to look for some review of the position and decision once the period was up as there was, they said, sometimes a tendency to let it drift. Here the senior nurses are well aware of the moral positions being put forward for the various views held and yet have to manage the clinical practicalities. This is a clear example of the utility of an analysis of the social context when we try to make sense of the moral dimension of intensive care.

The ways in which experienced senior nursing staff nudged along the process of making the decision to withdraw are illustrated in an extract from an interview with two senior nurses. They provided a rich seam of data as they were experienced long standing colleagues and spurred one another on in our discussion. They are talking about their feelings of frustration when they have to continue aggressive intensive care when all the signs suggest that withdrawal would be the preferred option (Melia 2001).

> *WG*: I felt that a bit with the other patient, Mr C, I felt very much like that with him. I felt I was pushing a bit and getting a lot of disinterest in a way, or like 'what is the point?' It is an inevitable thing, 'stop worrying about his platelets and stop worrying about ...'
>
> *MV*: But that was the thing about him, he was one of these patients that probably was never going to survive.
>
> *WG*: Yes, probably he should have died the weekend I had him but a doctor chose to resuscitate him and he was on huge amount of drugs and ...
>
> *MV*: But until you are told not to, that's what I found so frustrating with that. There was never a documented order from that consultant, not to resuscitate this man. So every time like either I was there on part of or certainly a shift I was doing whatever I could for any patient that was under my care. Then I was getting this apathetic sort of looks at the ward round like, well what are you trying to achieve here? Because it looks like it was an inevitable outcome.
>
> *WG*: But it was horrible wasn't it?
>
> *MV*: Well I think that was the worst thing, we ...
>
> *WG*: Yes, we discussed that quite a lot outside work the two of us, because we were on opposite shifts at the time.
>
> *MV*: It was also hard about the day he died you know 9 a.m. and he was just falling to bits and bleeding everywhere, his blood pressure was no good and terrible and the consultant on the ward round said no we have to do everything. I said right OK, I am going to be on your back every second of this morning and every second of the day, because I am fed up of every doctor saying that to me. I said you do half-heartedness and then you just walk away and leave him and nobody does anything, so I will be on your back every five seconds about what is happening to this man – 'his BP is still low, his BP is still low, his BP is still low' – because I had got it up to here because it was the same every day you know, oh well we have just got to keep going but, to me, he was dead. You know he was physically dead.

This distinction between the observable reality 'physically dead' and the physiological indicators – cardiac output, blood pressure and so on – is well described by Seymour (2000). Seymour notes how physicians

> negotiate a 'natural death' in intensive care by means of complex interactional strategies in which the timing of treatment withdrawal is carefully planned, and is accompanied by expressions of

belief about the causation of death. (2000: 103)

She talks of 'bodily dying' and 'technical dying' and argues that these must be 'aligned' in order for death to occur at the 'right' time. Containing and preventing divergence between bodily and technical dying are represented as the basis of 'nature taking its course' and 'natural death' in intensive care (2000: 103).

It is this kind of situation that the cardiac surgery nurses in the ethics study described. Their rather harrowing account, whilst not common, was not atypical (Melia 2001). It gives a very clear picture of the different perspectives of the health care professionals involved in intensive care. This account is an example of another feature of the prolonged decision to withdraw, that is when nurses perceive medical staff to be drawing back from the situation, leaving the nurses feeling rather isolated. When the doctors stepped back there was a sense that the care really had become clinically, and very probably morally, futile. In these situations the moral dimension of intensive care is very evident. The frustration expressed by the nurses in the cardiac unit in the above extract stems from the mismatch of the moral position and the continuing of treatment.

Interestingly one insight that this analysis offers is that nurses adopt a moral position with regard to surgeons' behaviour when treatment is withdrawn, or its withdrawal is imminent. The doctors most likely to 'walk away' are the surgeons: once they can do no more they pull out. The reaction of the nurses is understandable on one analysis and unreasonable on another. As the nurses see it, the surgeons have undermined the work of the ICU. This has a subtle effect on the legitimation of the ICU. It is as if intensive care cannot somehow be critical without the high profile involvement of doctors (Melia 2001). The British Medical Association publication refers to the fact that 'Many nurses have reported concern about what they perceive as "moral distancing" on the part of some doctors' (1999: 45). Walby et al. describe a similar situation when 'visiting consultants' as opposed to the ICU consultant in charge 'will insist on mounting treatment when the unit nursing staff are convinced that there is no hope, and nurses feel that this view is shared by the ICU consultant' (1994: 38).

This is an example of the organisation of the hospital having a part in the shaping of decisions. Anspach (1987) makes the point in the context of her study of neonatal intensive care. She describes an 'ecology of knowledge' in the unit with different professions construing the 'facts' in different ways and arriving at different interpretations and views on prognosis: 'the newborn ICU *qua* organisation allocates different types of information to those who work within it, and, in so doing, defines the character of the data that each group brings to the life and death decision' (1987: 217). Anspach says that it became apparent that there was a pattern to the conflicts between nurses and physicians: 'most often it was nurses, and, less frequently, the residents who were the first to conclude that the infant would not recover' (1987: 217).

Returning to the cardiac surgery ICU discussion, the main concern of the research with intensive care nurses was to gain an understanding of the ethical issues in intensive care and to combine moral philosophical and sociological analysis to that end (Melia 2001). The nurses' somewhat judgemental view on the doctors 'standing back' or 'moral distancing' when treatment becomes futile is an example of the importance of an understanding of the social context within which moral positions are taken up.

The nurses convey in their descriptions of looking after intensive care patients a strong sense of the need for team decisions and consensus. Even when this was not the reality, there was a lot of reference to the fact that consensus was the ideal situation and that the temporary loss of that state should not be taken as an indication that teamwork was in decline. This is evidenced in one nurse's comments during a discussion of how differences of opinion are handled in the ICU:

the consultants are very open and they do ask the nurse's opinion at the bedside, they do appreciate that they are the ones that are there for the twelve and a half hours, not the one that makes the decision and walks away and leaves it to happen ... It is not good all the time, we are all human beings, but I do think that if the nurses are unhappy about what has happened it is usually aired.

Given the imbalance of power and autonomy between medicine and nursing, Downie notes that '[nurses] are increasingly demanding consultation before important decisions affecting patient care are taken' (1996: 4). He goes on to say that 'group decision-making involves group responsibility. If the nursing profession wants an equal claim to be heard, then nurses must be willing to be held responsible for their decisions' (1996: 4).

The success of intensive care is as much contingent upon the nursing input as it is upon the medical and, most important of all, it relies upon co-operative working between nursing and medicine. Downie's exhortation is practical and ethical, rather than legal, for it remains the case that decisions about diagnosis and treatment are medical decisions. Nurses are clearly responsible and accountable at law for their own actions; they are not, though, legally responsible for taking decisions to continue or withdraw treatment. However, Downie's point is pertinent because nurses do, as he says, make their views known. These data suggest that doctors and nurses recognise where the authority and responsibility for the decision to withhold or withdraw treatment lies, but equally well recognise the need for co-operation in the ICU (Melia 2001). Consensus, whilst not a requirement at law, is given prominence and is thought to be highly desirable as a means of preserving teamwork. It is as much a moral solidarity as anything that is sought. The main threat to the integrity of the team emanates from differences of opinion around the withdrawal of treatment. As one senior sister put it, 'the only break-down in relations in the multidisciplinary team comes when junior staff who are with the patient all the time cannot see the consultant's point of view' (Melia 2001). Interestingly she also commented that the situation is often worse for the junior medical staff, who also spend a lot of their time on the unit and close to patients, because they are less experienced in intensive care than are some of the nursing staff at the bedside.

As we saw, the intensive care nurses expressed some concerns when the surgeons backed away from a case. In so doing the legitimacy of the ICU appeared in the nurses' view to be compromised. Seymour discuss-es the 'problematic constitution of "nursing care only" within intensive care' (2000: 106). She notes that as the technological means of 'reading the body' have developed this has tended to cause doctors to 'bolster the legitimacy of *technical dying* over and above *bodily dying*' (2000: 126).

COLLECTIVE RESPONSIBILITY IN THE ICU

It could be argued that medicine is organisationally bound to remain overtly involved in intensive care, even when the medical role has been overtaken by the process of withdrawal of treatment or awaiting death, to ensure that the team holds together. Collective responsibility works in the interests of the smooth functioning of the ICU. In a sense it has to prevail as if it were a requirement, not a legal but a moral requirement. The sociological analysis of the interviews with ICU nurses (Melia 2001) sheds some light on the informal and unstated social organisation of the ICU. Whilst legally the responsibility for the clinical decisions lies with the anaesthetist in charge, the interdependence of medicine and nursing is such that the team works best when it proceeds as if there were col-lective moral responsibility for the decisions taken. Consensus is an important symbol and a crucial day to day working arrangement for ensuring the solidarity of the team and allowing it to move on, unscathed, from difficult clinical situations to face the next as a fully co-operative and collegial entity. Intensive care relies on the integrity of the team and the unfailing functioning of teamwork, and consequently this need is more important than are other temporary lapses in interprofes-sional relations and disagreements over treatment in individual cases. One central lesson to be drawn from the close study of ICU work is the importance of the team.

That the main issue confronting intensive care nurses raised in these interviews was the withdrawal of treatment is not remarkable (Melia 2001). The steady stream of cases in the law courts establishing the legal position on issues of futility and the limits of medical practice have left questions over the commencement of treatment and its withdrawal. Indeed the complex legal and ethical situation is such that the British Medical Association (1999) has published guidance for decision making in cases where withholding or withdrawing may be options. In this they make it clear that

> Although ultimately the responsibility for treatment decisions rests with the clinician in charge of the patient's care, it is important, where non-emergency decisions are made, that account is taken of the views of other health professionals involved in the patient's care and people close to the patient, in order to ensure that the decision is as well informed as possible. (1999: 45)

Withdrawal, as we have seen, is not a simple or a single act: it may take the form of continuing to ventilate but not to add anything new by way of other life support drugs, and so on. If 'withdrawal' has taken the form of 'add nothing new, but don't stop ventilating' then the patient is in something of a limbo state in the ICU, receiving intensive care but not in its full sense. Jennett says that

> Nursing staff in intensive care units are geared to making all efforts to sustain life ... It is, however, often difficult for the staff to scale down the level of care when this becomes appropriate because there is no longer any prospect of a favourable outcome. (1994: 870)

This is the same point that Seymour (2000) makes in her discussion of 'nursing care only' in the ICU. She sums it up neatly when she writes of 'the complexity and sheer paradoxicality that attend the delivery of nursing care to dying people in intensive care'.

When the nursing staff are shouldering more of the intensive care than are the medical staff, there is potential for dissent in the team. It could be said to be surprising that in situations where the treatment was halted and nursing care was the main activity, this did not always go down well with the nurses. After all, the complaint is often about a lack of independence of medicine. Several nurses during interview expressed the view that they felt a sense of being 'left with it' when there was no further medical interest taken in the management of a patient (Melia 2001). The feeling of being 'left with it', which some nurses expressed when medical staff, surgeons in all cases, stood back, was not entirely rational. These nurses acknowledged that it was perfectly reasonable, but only up to a point, for surgeons to stand back when there was no more for them to do. However, the nurses felt that in so doing the surgeons conveyed a sense of futility and so undermined the intensive care work, albeit intensive care nursing only, that went on in their absence, as it were. Ironically, these nurses were likely to be the ones who quibbled when decisions about withdrawal of treatment were prolonged or postponed. The irony is that nurses want to be included in the decisions which technically, legally even, are not theirs to make, yet they feel abandoned when medical staff back off and leave them to the part of the work which is properly the province of nursing. This can be explained through an understanding of the work organisation. Medicine's withdrawal from the scene comes across in the nurses' accounts as a ratcheting down of care such that it is no longer 'intensive' in the usual sense. This emphasises the point that intensive care has to be a team effort.

THE IMPORTANCE OF TEAMWORK IN THE ICU

It is arguable that the 'nursing only' dilemma, that is the situation where it is no longer sensible for the patient to stay in ICU but where death is not imminent, is really a question of moving the patient out of intensive care. In this case the 'moving out' question is a pale imitation of the initial hard question of moving in, of admitting. To move a patient out of ICU seems to be disruptive and rather like a ratcheting down of service, yet to allow the patient to stay is a misuse of resources. To retain a patient in ICU beyond the time where there is benefit to be gained can lead to a potential for deprivation of others. If a bed is suddenly needed, the transfer out of the patient can take place in an unseemly hurry and constitute poor practice. Stay and see is similar to admit and see. Morally the question of when to move is reasonably clear, but in the messy clinical reality, which the sociological analysis shows up so well, it is a very understandable line of argument that a patient should remain in ICU if at all possible for reasons of pleasing the family and not appearing to be insensitive. Seymour says, on the basis of her fieldwork:

> While companions understood the need for transfer, they expressed regret at losing the attentive nursing care that intensive care could provide to the dying person, and the emotional support they had gained from the formation of close relationships with the nurses primarily responsible for the patient. (2000: 162)

One of the attractions of working in intensive care has to do with what was described as the 'buzz'; also the variety of cases and a sense of working at the cutting edge. For this incentive to prevail, the whole team is needed. Surgeons 'standing back' and even, as one nurse put it, 'getting bored' is a sign that the 'buzz' of the ICU has gone. The nurses' message seemed to be that the team has to stick together even when no other role remains for the medics beyond that of moral support for the nurses and relatives who are still carrying out their roles. It is very probable that the nurses actually shared the surgeons' sense of futility, but were not able to stand back until the decision to withdraw had been made. So whilst the earlier interview discussion between the two senior nurses at first

appears to be a frank criticism of the medical staff, it is rather more subtle than that. It is an expression of the frustrations experienced by the
team members, who, whilst they are fully engaged in patient care, do not
bear the practical or legal responsibility for making the decisions. The
nurses in the intensive care team who generally draw strength from
knowing that all members are pulling together come under pressure in
these circumstances. This puts the team itself under strain because the
issues in question are not simply organisational and matters of professional status, but complex moral questions. They are the moral questions
which are embedded in the social organisation of intensive care work
(Melia 2001).

Seymour argues that it is the nurses that allow the team to continue
despite differences of opinion as they do not criticise openly. She says
this is because nurses recognise that medical staff are effectively constrained against basing their action on anything other than technological
data. Seymour also notes that nurses accept that 'the technological
recognition of dying *lags behind* the acknowledgement of that state as a
material fact' (2000: 156).

One of the main concerns is to ensure that there is no direct
causative link between the withdrawal of treatment and the death. The
body has to be defined as being no longer able to take advantage of medical technology. In this chapter we have started to make the case for col-
legiality in health care and health care ethics. The main point is that
whilst nurses have little say about whether to admit a patient to ICU,
they are involved more in decisions about withdrawal. It would seem to
be the case that a little more understanding of the different perspectives
that the professions of medicine and nursing take would ease tensions.

Much of the day to day practice of intensive care has to do with
effecting clinical possibilities in socially acceptable ways. The health care
team has to work with the law and in ways which are acceptable to the
patients' relatives. In the UK the law is clear that it is the medical consultant in charge of the care who is responsible for the decision, but the
views of other health professions, and of patients (where possible) or of
relatives, have to be sought. It is sometimes the case that when the views
of relatives are sought, they misunderstand and assume that the decision
is theirs to take (Melia 2001). Zussman (1992: 101) says that in the USA
the patients' rights are not in dispute and physicians recognise these
rights, *but* they want to reserve some of the decisions to themselves, as
matters of technique. The question becomes one of where the boundaries
lie between matters of value (ethics) and matters of technical knowledge.
Zussman (1992: 101) notes that the sociologist's interest in ICU lies in the
drama of the efforts of the doctors to maintain their discretion in decisions concerning life and death. The discretion that doctors seek to retain
is mostly used to limit treatment – hence the debate with law and ethics.

Knowing when to stop is clearly an issue in the ICU. We have seen that there are differences of opinion about when aggressive treatment becomes futile, with nurses and doctors sometimes taking different standpoints on this. Also, we noted that surgeons and anaesthetists in charge of the ICU can have difficulty in arriving at an agreement on when it is wise to continue with treatment. In many ways this comes back to the question of the proper use of the intensive care unit. Even when there is an agreement to stop treatment, there can still be difficulties in terms of where the patient should be nursed. If they require 'nursing care only' then, comfortable and well staffed though it may be in the view of the relatives, the ICU is not the place for the dying patient. When the nurses complain that by stepping back from care the surgeons undermine intensive care, they are right: intensive care is a multidisciplinary effort which has its place as long as there is some prospect of success. When this is no longer the case the patient should be transferred to a more suitable environment. Questions of the use of resources and the readiness of ICU beds are relevant here. It might appear to be a little unseemly to move a patient out of ICU once they are not being offered the full range of care on offer there. However, if the ready availability of beds is an important feature of the intensive care service, the transfer out of patients who are not benefiting from intensive care is a necessary evil in the system. In the next chapter the theme of the proper use of intensive care is developed.

NOTES

1   Never having liked this expression I will use the term 'relative' to refer to family and friends representing the patient's interests. I do so on the grounds that friends are related by friendship whereas family need not imply friend.

2   A reference to the popular quiz show 'Mastermind' hosted by Magnus Magnusson, where the rules say that if a question has started before the time up signal, it is finished. Magnusson always says, 'I've started so I'll finish.'

3   *Re Quinlan* 335 A2d 647 1976, 70 NJ 10 (1976).

4   *Airedale NHS Trust* v. *Bland* [1993] 1 All ER 821; *Law Hospital NHS Trust* v. *Lord Advocate* [1996] SLT 848.

iii the palliation–care–cure triangle

THE PATIENT'S BEST INTERESTS

The central aim of both nursing and medicine is to act in the best interests of the patient. This is such an obvious statement that it is hardly
worth setting down on the page. However, the old adage 'easier said
than done' springs readily to mind once we begin to think out the practicalities of acting in the patient's best interests. Most difficult, perhaps,
is the thorny question of how we know what the patient would say these
are: the question is complex. The place of advance directives is relevant
here as they present a very clear example of situations where the
patient's interests are known, yet they still lead to complex discussions
about the validity of the patient's view on their situation. The problem is
that consultants in charge of the case have to be sure that the circumstances they face are the ones anticipated by the patient when the
advance directive was made.

   The British Medical Association (1995) specifically uses the term
'advance directive' for a refusal of treatment made by a person when
they were fully capable of taking an informed decision. The whole area
of advance directives, or 'living wills' as they are also known, is complicated by the fact that the question of what is being refused and under
what circumstances is by no means straightforward. The BMA Code of
Practice with respect to advance directives discusses the various forms
that the statements of preferred treatment can take. These statements in
certain circumstances have legal force. An advance refusal of treatment
is as valid as a refusal of treatment that any competent, informed person
might make for themselves in the course of their illness. The difficulty
which the advance nature of the expression of choice introduces is the
need to ensure that the circumstances in which it has to be acted upon
are those envisaged when the statement was made. The clinicians
involved may well opt to take legal advice before following a patient's

wishes as expressed in an advance directive. This need not be seen as the old spectre of medical paternalism arising again; rather it is evidence of the shift that we are seeing towards patient-centred care and a health care system which increasingly involves the law. As Zussman (1992) has noted, the decline in the power of medicine and the move towards a greater concern for patients' rights and wishes have brought with them an increased role for the law in the sphere of health care practice. This of course does not remove the need for clinical judgements to be made by clinicians – clinical judgements which are in part moral judgements.

Boyd, in the course of an interesting paper on the ethical implications of advance directives, makes the point that what patients most fear is 'the possibility not of cancer (unless it affects the brain) but conditions such as stroke, dementia and degenerative disease' and that it is 'degradation and indignity' that they fear more than death. In other words, in the use of the advance directive patients are looking to secure a good death (1999: 5). Boyd notes that there is nothing ethically contentious about the patient requesting that they are 'not kept alive by extraordinary or disproportionate means'. However, he points out that this question is only part of the picture. There remains the question of how to ensure that a patient's expectations are realised when their quality of life is such that they would not wish to continue.

We have to accept that there are now many areas of medicine where the question of best interests is rendered difficult either because of the range of technological possibilities on offer or because the social context has, in developed countries at least, altered such that 'life at any cost' has become a rather prominent position. It was noted in a number of the interviews that I undertook with ICU nurses that people do hold rather contradictory views about what they think should happen in difficult end-of-life situations. People may hold the view, 'I wouldn't like to be left in that situation', when they contemplate the condition of someone in persistent vegetative state (PVS) or with what they would regard as a very poor quality of life; at the same time they will demand that 'everything be done' for their relatives.

Zussman (1992) in his study of ICU makes the point that physicians often felt constrained by the law. The President's Commission (1982) made it clear that 'final authority' for decisions to withhold treatment is the patient's. This extract from Zussman's presentation of fieldnotes in his work makes the point: the ICU staff are debating the question of whether to follow the wishes of the sister of a patient whose prospects are poor and they think that dialysis will be futile.

'She wants to prolong this state. We're saying it's not worth preserving.' 'And that,' she continued, 'is not a "medical issue".' 'I wish,' she concluded, 'the family didn't have the final say. But ... they do.' (1992: 178)

The British Medical Association (1995) Code of Practice in relation to advance directives makes it clear that doctors cannot be legally bound through such statements to embark upon treatments which they feel are futile or inappropriate. Also, the Code includes the principle that basic care should not be refused through either advance directive or the instruction of an advocate to make such a request on the patient's behalf. The provision of basic needs through nursing care includes food and drink, but does not extend to artificial means of providing this.

Thus the main problem with the advance directive, and more so with the not for resuscitation (NFR) order, is the specificity of the request. The palliative care literature is of some help here. Randall and Downie (1996), palliative care consultant and philosopher respectively, provide a useful discussion of obligatory and optional treatments in the context of palliative care. Here they raise the question of the benefits of providing hydration by artificial means as a palliative measure. This question of the simple provision of water provokes emotional responses especially among nurses who have day to day care of patients who are semi-conscious or unconscious. Although the provision of water is such a basic need, it may distress a patient who is near death. Randall and Downie say:

> at present we simply do not know whether these patients are dis-
> tressed by thirst or not, we do not know how great the risk of fluid
> overload is, or whether poor or absent fluid intake significantly
> alters the course of the disease. (1996: 123)

Neither do we know, they go on to say, whether hydration is burden-some, and so

> it is not possible to make a judgement about whether hydration in
> this circumstance is morally obligatory or optional. (1996: 124)

Randall and Downie make the point that to undertake such research would in itself be ethically difficult. But the fact remains that until we know whether artificial hydration helps or merely prolongs dying or actually causes distress, clinicians are left with difficult clinical judge-ments to make in these circumstances.

Intensive care is the most obvious area of medicine where the imperative to do something in order that life will continue is particular-ly strong. As we saw in the last chapter, the culture of the ICU is strong-ly proactive and it is often quite a struggle to decide to withdraw treat-ment once all the stops have been pulled out to treat. Given the range of treatment options available in oncology the same ethical question exists there. Also, in the area of palliative care the extent and effects of treat-ment are varied. As Randall and Downie put it, 'Whilst palliative treat-ments are given primarily either to prolong life or to relieve suffering or disability, the effects of many treatments are mixed' (1996: 109).

The theme of this chapter is a concern with the ethical issues which arise in a consideration of the different approaches to the management of disease. These approaches can be presented as the straightforward aim to cure, the palliative approach and the decision to settle for 'nursing care only'. I have characterised these approaches as a triangle with the sides representing cure, palliation and care, in order to show that the three are not unrelated. In order to explore the complexities involved here I have set down three reasonably distinct approaches to the treatment or case management of the patient, whilst recognising that the clinical and social realities are complicated. Theoretically these can be presented as clear-cut entities, yet practically, as we might imagine, they are not so distinct. A little arbitrariness, at least in the first instance, may help to clarify the debate.

INTERRELATIONSHIP BETWEEN PALLIATION, CARE AND CURE

The relationship between care, cure and palliation first struck me as an important area for ethical debate when I had a close personal experience of someone undergoing aggressive surgical treatment for cancer. The surgery was clearly intended to be curative, so at the very least the outcome could have been to have bought time. It could not be described as palliative as the rhetoric of the surgeons was of cure within the meanings of that term in the context of cancer. The burden of the treatment was such that at times it was difficult to construe the management of this case in terms of care. Caring certainly went on, but not in any sense of 'nursing care only', or 'terminal care', since the intervention was intended to produce something akin to cure.

At that time I began to think in general terms about the original intentions and the ultimate outcome, and about how things can turn out unexpectedly. If the intention was to effect a cure or a remission and it failed, was the patient in some ways in a worse position than if such an approach had not been adopted in the first place? Might a palliative approach have been a better option in the long run? Hovering over this discussion is the perennial problem of uncertainty: 'if I knew then what I know now' is not an attitude usefully adopted in medicine where uncertainty comes with the territory. Moral debates conducted in consequentialist terms often founder on the lack of predictability in clinical judgements.

Along similar lines I also wondered about the question of starting out with one intention and in the event coming closer to another outcome than had been expected. Does, for instance, palliative care ever cross over into being close to cure or remission but not close enough? Would then 'nursing care only' or 'terminal care' have been a better

option? This set of theoretical possibilities is completed by a consideration of the possible situation where there is a giving up on cure or palliation in favour of care. On the occasions that this move from cure to care
happens in the ICU it is in very sharp contrast to the usual proactive
approach. The move sometimes takes a while to effect.

In my study, one interview with two intensive care nurses makes
this point well:

> *VH*: ... a 40-year-old who had been with us a month, she had a
> double valve replacement and never got better, her tricuspid valve
> failed after the aortic and mitral were replaced and she became
> critically ill for like 2–3 weeks and the decision was always to oper-
> ate or not and try and fix the tricuspid, would she survive surgery,
> and that went on and on and on and eventually they got to the
> stage that they did decide to, with the discussion with the family,
> they were advised that she probably wouldn't survive and maybe
> this is the end of the road, but no they wanted this one shot at sur-
> gery so they did do it and she had terrible problems with bleeding
> after and dreadful liver failure when she went in for surgery, so
> pretty hopeless really, so that there was like a bit of a battle for
> two days, and BTS [Blood Transfusion Service] were extremely
> good, but I think at the end of the day everybody realised as much
> blood as we gave it wasn't going to make a difference and she
> wasn't going to survive. And it was really distressing because
> there then became, I felt a little bit of, it is terrible to say, but bore-
> dom from the medical staff but because I think we have a lot of
> surgeons around, surgically there was nothing more to do, so she
> suddenly didn't become their problem so much in a way or as
> interesting in a way. We do have anaesthetists that cover, we did-
> n't used to have, whoever was on covered the ICU, but we now
> have a consultant doing a week at a time.
> *KM*: Ah right, and the others do the anaesthetics.
> *GR*: Yes, so it actually took me in the unit to go and find this con-
> sultant to explain the situation and to discuss what we could do
> about it, because it really was very distressing, she had young
> daughters of 13, 14 who were having to see their mother you
> know in that state it was really awful. But I think the whole point
> that I found most upsetting about it was that although the medical
> staff, as I say, the surgeons, there was nothing more they could
> do, but there didn't seem to be a senior anaesthetist, intensivist,
> that was sort of around, so anyway we contacted the consultant
> surgeon and with the anaesthetist we decided that it was time to
> withdraw treatment. So we did it very quickly, within ten minutes
> we completely withdrew treatment and gave some sedation.

The difficulty of moving from the highly technologised approach to the
cure to the business of treating symptoms and providing care has in part
to do with the need for a change in emphasis. That is to say, in the high-

est of high tech environments the health care professionals are always concerned with care; it does however have to find a place amid the technologically driven work. Seymour puts this well when she says that what happens is the relocation of death and dying 'from the biomedical sphere to the arena of emotion and familial intimacy' (2000: 106). Ashby notes that unless there is a better understanding of end-of-life care the options on offer will be the

> abrupt cessation of treatment, minimalist palliative care and treatment directed at bringing about a rapid dying process, to excessive caution about being seen to be instrumental in causing the death. (1998: 74)

The debates about what strategy or approach to adopt in each case share some similarities with the ICU questions about withholding treatment. If palliative care is the preferred option when the offerings of the oncology services are deemed to be too burdensome or are unlikely to produce the desired results, there is a need for a transition to 'nursing care only'. This hesitation is similar to that which is found in withdrawal situations in ICU.

Clark and Seymour say that 'palliative care is the active total care of patients whose disease is not responsive to curative treatment' (1999: 83). There has been considerable debate around terminology in palliative care, with distinctions being made between palliative care and terminal care and difficulties being raised when the focus on the one detracts from the meaning of the other. Biswas says that 'palliative care shifts the focus of attention away from death' (1999: 135). This is in much the same way as I am suggesting that the cure and palliative sides of the triangle shift the focus away from care.

By including terminal care as an important part of palliative care the National Council for Hospice and Specialist Palliative Care Services (NCHSPCS 1995) makes a useful contribution to the debate, yet it also raises other questions about where the line is crossed from palliative to terminal. The World Health Organisation (1990), in a report concerned with pain relief in cancer and palliative care, stated that there need not be such a sharp division between curative treatment and palliative care. The one should phase into and include the other as circumstances dictate.

The difficulties in distinguishing between the definitions of palliative care and terminal care, and indeed the nature of the interface between curative treatment and palliative care, stem in part from the randomised controlled trials (RCTs) in cancer cure. These trials are seen as the gold standard by which medical advances in research are made. The main problem with them is that they focus on length of survival. This being the case, the label 'terminal care' can carry negative connotations for some (Ahmedzai 1996; Doyle et al. 1993; Higginson 1993).

If we are to consider the ethical aspects of this area of health care, we need to focus on the purpose of the care – be it curative, palliative or terminal – as the important factor. In other words the focus needs to be on what the intention is, what the clinicians are trying to achieve when they adopt care, cure or palliation as their approach to the management of a particular patient. The measurements of outcomes of treatments cannot be in years of survival alone. The quality of life is a rather clichéd expression; nonetheless issues of quality have to enter into the clinical decisions about moving from cure to palliative or terminal care. As the transition is made the aims have to be clear as they will also change: achieving a longer survival time is of no use if it is merely delaying death. So the goal of a curative treatment with its success measured in an RCT by the number of years survived is clearly to add years to life. The goal of palliative care may be to prolong life or to relieve symptoms: the effects are often mixed.

Randall and Downie (1996) provide a good discussion of treatments available in palliative care. They reject the commonly made division of health care activity into medical treatment (often described as cure) and treatments which can be described as care. They say it is then often assumed that medical treatments are always optional whilst care is always obligatory. They prefer to 'take the view that any palliative care activity may be either appropriate or inappropriate' (1996: 111).

They have sound reasons for taking this morally neutral stance on treatments *per se*. First, they argue that it is difficult to determine whether some treatments should be designated medical or nursing, for example artificial feeding. They also note, and here I would strongly agree, that such a division

> encourages doctors and nurses to see themselves in two separate camps, because there is a general understanding that doctors are responsible for medical treatment whereas nurses are responsible for care. The division of roles does not encourage professional partnership and teamwork. (1996: 110)

Their last reason for rejecting the 'medical treatment is optional whilst nursing care is obligatory' position is that the dichotomy suggests that whilst medical intervention may or may not be helpful, nursing care will always be helpful and, perhaps more to their point, never harmful. Their example makes the point well:

> the nursing care option of aggressive management of pressure sores involving debridement and desloughing is not obligatory when the patient is comatose or imminently dying. Indeed, it is probably obligatory not to provide such care in this situation, but instead to pursue the less aggressive options of a sophisticated pressure-releasing mattress and dressings involving minimal disturbance. (1996: 110)

They go on to make the same point about artificial feeding in this situation, noting that 'any consideration of whether it may be best described as a medical treatment or nursing care is simply irrelevant' (1996: 110).

Palliative care occupies an interesting middle ground between aggressive curative treatment and nursing care only. Seymour (2000) notes that palliative care and intensive care are fields of health care which were developing at the same time in history. She says that palliative care has developed 'a reputation of avoiding overly interventionist treatments and of offering a range of "low-tech" options to people dying with advanced disease' (2000: 1).

Palliative care is traditionally seen as part of cancer care, although there are debates around the question of widening its scope. From the outset it was never intended that hospice and palliative care should remain associated only with oncology; the aim was that it should apply throughout medicine. Seymour suggests that those who might benefit from palliative care may be channelled down the wrong route, the aggressive intensive care route, because of the way that disease labels function. More specifically she says that because hospice and palliative care were initially developed for those dying from cancer, other groups of patients can be overlooked.

Palliative care, as we have seen, can be at times proactive; this could cause a lack of focus on care, or what is often referred to as *nursing care only*. The question for the health care professionals is whether to treat with the sole aim of making the patient comfortable (palliatively) or to treat more aggressively, that is working towards remission or as near to cure as is possible. The decision is not often straightforward and is likely to entail movement between one mode and another. Treatment with a view to effecting a cure is different from that directed towards palliation and in either case care may be compromised along the way.

Again Randall and Downie (1996) provide a good example. In the context of discussing the care of someone with cancer of the head and neck, they say: 'If a patient develops dysphagia (difficulty in swallowing) and tube-feeding by gastrostomy is undertaken, then that patient is likely to live long enough to develop either tracheal obstruction or haemorrhage' (1996: 118). They discuss other conditions, for example cervical cancer, where fairly simple low-risk palliative procedures can avert death by renal failure, only to allow the patient to live on to die a rather more unpleasant death from the more advanced pathology of the cancer. The renal failure option might be regarded as 'nature's way out', and an intervention by modern medicine can only hope to secure a delaying of death and, very probably, a less acceptable mode of death.

These circumstances call for fine clinical judgements – judgements which have a distinct moral content, especially when we consider the principles of informed consent and respect for persons. Patients have a right to know about their condition, but they also have a right not to exercise that right. This calls for especially sensitive judgements on the part of all health care professionals as they tread the line between accusations of paternalistic behaviour and not paying due attention to the autonomy of the individual. Treading this line may involve having what Randall and Downie refer to as 'a rather gruesome discussion about ways of dying' (1996: 118). These difficult areas also demand a co-ordinated approach from those caring for the patient. Teamwork and a shared, well debated view of the moral dimension of the decisions taken are essential if the fine clinical judgements are going to be carried through.

CONSEQUENCES – INTENDED AND UNINTENDED

The sides of the cure–care–palliation triangle are related, and a push in one direction has consequences in another. A decision to give nursing care only may overlook the cure potential if the main concern is for a non-aggressive, conservative approach to the management of the case. In such a scenario the end of life may be close at hand, but it would also be tranquil, and occur in surroundings where the ethos was to effect – to use a rather over-worked phrase – a good death. As we saw in the last chapter, the good death in the ICU is possible but difficult. Moreover, because the culture of the intensive care unit is necessarily one of proaction and aggressive treatment, when this is no longer appropriate the gear shift to other strategies tends to be regarded in negative terms. Giving up or backing off are the terms used by nurses to describe the standing back which medical staff tend to employ when there is no more for them to do.

Zussman (1992) notes with concern that he observed medical staff expressing the wish to abandon patients when they could not cure them. He says that even when the decision is not to continue with intensive care, it is rarely the case that all treatment ceases. Not for resuscitation (NFR) orders are, as we have noted, very closely circumscribed and involve cardio-pulmonary function. This leaves a good number of other circumstances where proactive treatment is perhaps not the best option, yet it is followed. Nature left to her own devices, as we noted above, is not always a sure route to a tranquil death. Particularly rampant cancers, if left unchecked, can be overwhelming: Randall and Downie make this point well.

In the 1980s I was a visiting ethics scholar in Perth, Western Australia. During a workshop for oncology nurses, the discussion turned to the rather radical pre-operative care and treatment that entailed women undergoing total pelvic clearance. This was undertaken with the patients' informed consent as a palliative measure in ovarian cancer. The nurses thought that it was barbaric and inhumane and they gave the surgeons a very hard time over this whenever there was an opportunity for discussion. In the workshops we got around to discussing the alternatives: mother nature is neither kinder nor less radical than the surgery when it comes to a frank consideration of unchecked ovarian cancer. The nurses gave the impression that they had the patients' interests at heart, implying that the doctors did not. The evidence for this view was that the surgeons were carrying out this very drastic surgery (the kind of thing that is known in the trade as horrendoplasty) and embroiling the nurses in this work through the pre-operative preparation, which involved total gut lavage. It was only after some very frank discussion, and with the surgeons showing some pathology slides detailing the result when nature was left to her own devices, and pointing out that the women had choice in the matter, that the nurses conceded the point and moved to a more collegial position.

Randall and Downie have a comment which would have been useful in those Australian workshops:

> a mother with young children will often accept life which she and others would consider to be of poor quality, because she knows that it is of great value to her family and therefore to her. Young women in this situation as the result of advanced malignant disease tend to be tenacious of life and want it prolonged in order to give them more time with their families. (1996: 120)

Palliative measures, including what may be regarded as radical and major surgery in the circumstances, can be justified if the benefits, albeit that they are short term, outweigh the disadvantages of nature taking her course. *Aggressive palliation*, if such a term can be used, could be thought of as 'near cure' or even 'failed cure'. In other words, aggressive measures can be countenanced when the outcome justifies it, as in the case of remission or cure. What is less clear is whether burdensome treatments can be justified on palliative grounds. The worry might be that an excessive focusing on the cure, or palliative treatment, could detract from a more care-oriented approach to the patient. If for example fairly radical surgery is undertaken in order to alleviate the symptoms of cancer (e.g. liver resection), the aim is palliation. The approach may appear to be more akin to that taken to effect a cure, and hence the notion of care may be lost amid the burden of the treatment. The overall aims of palliation are consistent with care, but the alleviation of symptoms may involve treatment which in another context would effect a cure.

Perhaps the best commentary on this kind of dilemma is Randall and Downie's view that palliative treatments or care should be judged on the basis of individual circumstances rather than having a situation where some are regarded as helpful measures and others not necessarily so. They say that it is sometimes morally justifiable not to offer life-prolonging or life-sustaining treatments to patients even though they are able to discuss them in a fully autonomous way. Such circumstances include when the treatments are

> physiologically futile, when their burden and risks greatly out-
> weigh their benefits, where they may prolong life so that much
> more unpleasant events which the patient declines to contem-
> plate or discuss are very likely to ensue. (1996: 120)

As we saw in Chapter 2, in the context of making decisions to withdraw treatment, the uncertainty which characterises medicine is the main difficulty when we try to work out what truly is in the patients' best interests. To bring about, by palliation, a continuation of life but not life of a quality that is desirable, suggests that to fall between the care and the cure sides of the triangle might be the unfortunate outcome of palliation.

So far I have attempted to show how doing one thing, be it caring, curing or palliating, can have unintended consequences. It might also be that the care which could be offered is compromised because of the emphasis being on cure or palliation. Put simply, the argument is that palliation which is too proactive or as it were 'aggressive palliation' could tip over to resemble an all-out approach to cure. The problem would lie in the fact that there would be no cure. In the theoretical terms of the care–cure–palliation triangle what I have termed 'aggressive palliation' could be represented as an action which overshot or went beyond the realms of palliation but then went on to stop short of cure.

The point at issue may be as much to do with the social organisation of these practices of cure, palliation and care and the way in which the health care professionals view the work they are doing. We have noted that the moral philosopher's approach to what 'ought' to be done contrasts with the sociological analysis of how health care workers bring about the clinical management of individuals within the social context of professional health care.

SOCIAL CONTEXT AND PROFESSIONAL PERSPECTIVES

Anspach (1987) talks about life and death decisions being taken in the neonatal ICU from the standpoint of the sociology of knowledge. The professions approach the same patient and ethical situation in different ways, sometimes with different priorities. The different health care workers in the ICU have different perspectives because they work within different social contexts in terms of the knowledge that they have of the infants. On this analysis the physicians have a more technically oriented approach to the infants whilst nurses take a more social interactive view, as they have more prolonged contact with the babies and so have a sense of them as, albeit tiny, social actors. Again we see the social organisation of health care being brought into play and the type and duration of the interaction between health care worker and patient being drawn upon, here by the nurses, in order to make claims to particular knowledge of the patient.

A patient who is thought to be failing, that is to say not benefiting from what the intensive care has to offer, ultimately becomes a 'dying patient'. Depending upon the practicalities and the timescale of the patient's demise, the dying will occur in the ICU or in a ward. The atmosphere around patients becomes very clear to them if they are conscious. Their relatives too are aware of the ethos of the clinical setting: the action of the ICU compared with the peaceful and calming atmosphere of the hospice, the familiarity of home and so on. In one of her interviews with a family member of a man dying in ICU, Seymour notes that the family were impressed by the way that their relative was treated in the unit, saying that 'The nurses knew the same as I did that Jack wasn't going to come out of that coma, but they still treated him like a patient that was going to be alright' (2000: 46). This description of a patient as someone who was going to make it, to be alright, is a very telling comment on how lay people view hospitals and especially intensive care.

Much of this discussion comes back to the central issue of the proper use of the ICU, and similar debates which run on from that about the limits and appropriateness of health care treatment. The most difficult question is when to stop. Intensive care represents the dramatic end of the spectrum and, as we have seen, starts with the question of whether to offer intensive care in the first place. The decision is often to admit, even though a high percentage of patients do not survive either their stay in ICU or for many weeks after discharge. Once the first decision to treat has been taken then the next difficult question, if the prognosis is not good, is whether or not to stop treatment. At heart the question is the same: should treatment not take place, and is it time for nature to run her course?

Decisions have to be taken about when to stop attempting surgery, chemotherapy, radiotherapy, and eventually the question arises of moving to 'nursing care only'. Oncology offers such a range of possible treatment options, with second, third and more alternatives being tried if the first choice is not successful, that the temptation is to keep going, to try one more chemotherapy regime to see if it will produce a remission. As we have seen, these are similar problems to those experienced in the ICU. Having started out on the treatment with a view to cure or remission, it is difficult to withdraw. In a seminal paper, Jennett describes this difficulty as the 'vicious circle of commitment' (1984: 1709).

PROLONGING LIFE OR DELAYING DEATH

Depending upon individual circumstances it is sometimes difficult to know whether it is best to allow the inevitable to happen or to treat, such that the patient will arrive at a physiological state which is stable but in which the quality of life has to be questioned. Both intensive care and treatments which are often termed *unnatural means*, for example artificial feeding, can be seen as means of prolonging life or delaying death. The danger of both is that the technological imperative sometimes over-shadows the question of quality of life. The ICU is not the only setting where these difficult choices have to be made. The debates in the ICU are high profile and serve both in practice and in the literature to shape the issues, but the self-same dilemma of when to stop occurs in stroke units and care of the elderly. Following a cerebral vascular accident patients face a period of uncertainty when the outcome, particularly in terms of their level of impairment, is unknown. There are windows of opportunity along the way when decisions to feed (by parenteral or enteral means) are taken in order to allow the patient to regain the strength required to get through the period. Without artificial nutritional support they are very likely to fail. The same ethical questions arise in the ICU or near-intensive care where support is offered through feeding and nursing care, as opposed to the more typical ICU scenario where respiratory assistance is also needed. Either way, the treatment offered, be it higher or lower tech, can be regarded as a prolonger of life or delayer of death. If prolonging life merely delays death, there is little to be said for it. The central question is the quality of that life. It is a much debated topic in both medical and nursing ethics. Uncertainty again is a central feature of this state.

The use of permanently inserted tubes in the stomach (percutaneous endoscopic gastrostomy, PEG) to allow feeding raises ethical questions and particularly difficult questions about if and when to stop such treatment. One possible outcome of such life-sustaining approaches to treatment is that they are a means of prolonging life through to the next stroke which may bring with it more serious impairment. I am not suggesting that there are easy ways through this, but it is worth noting that the 'windows of opportunity' that present themselves, times when we might be wise not to act, have to be considered. Such windows can arise in areas other than ICU and may not present such a stark choice as does a not for resuscitation (NFR) order, but the consequences are as grave. The public imagination and the 'can do' attitude to what is possible in health care suggest unfettered progress, yet many would argue that the language of patients' rights causes health care workers to hold back (Zussman 1992).

The care–cure–palliation triangle is a way of representing in broad

terms the options in health care. The three are interrelated and shade
into one another. If there is too much emphasis upon one it can be to the
detriment of the patient as it draws attention away from another, potentially more apt, approach. It may be that flexibility is what is required,
an open approach to the options and a willingness to change according
to circumstances. In the ICU debates about withdrawal it seems that
things work out for the best when professionals are pulling together.
Teamwork is clearly the way forward, but it has to be remembered that
teamwork involves more than a number of disciplines being involved: it
requires that they work together. This interdependence of nursing and
medicine has evolved to the point where two professional groups understand and, by and large, respect one another's roles and professional
values. However, it remains the case that medicine has the dominant
position in health care, and it is the doctor who is responsible for and
ultimately carries the legal can for the patient's care. When medicine and
nursing come into conflict over treatment, provided there is no malprac-
tice in question, then it is legally and most often practically the case that
the medical view prevails.

Zussman (1992) discusses the differences between how medicine
and nursing work in the ICU and he characterises their behaviour in
terms of physicians 'doing physiology' whilst the nurses are doing the
'caring'. After reading his analysis one might be tempted to add 'carp-
ing' to the nurses' activities! Zussman's point is that medicine, as practised in the ICUs he observed, is more science and less personal care oriented. In the context of the discussion in this chapter this would place it
firmly on the 'cure' side of the triangle. Zussman says that patients disappear in ICU and return in the form of numbers, clinical parameters,
clinical chemistry results, blood gases and so on. He says that 'Intensive
care, in particular, is organised around a notion that medicine at its best
- at its most heroic, its purest - is about physiology and physiology
alone' (1992: 36).

Atkinson, writing some years after Zussman, makes similar points
in his analysis when he talks of 'reading the body', noting that 'in principle, every organ and every system may be inspected and sampled'
(1995: 61). The Foucauldian idea of the gaze can now, according to
Atkinson, be dispersed through to other departments in the hospital:

> The bedside remains as the original site of clinical understanding.
> It is to the bedside that the clinical investigation returns: it is visit-
> ed repeatedly by clinicians. But the space of the bedside does not
> bound the clinical gaze. The bedside itself becomes a site of data
> collection. The body is sampled, invaded, measured and inspect-
> ed, in order to yield images and information. Those data can then
> be scrutinised and interrogated elsewhere – in the specialist
> departments and laboratories of the modern hospital. (1995: 61)

This representation, a compelling one, of medicine's main functions of diagnosis and cure illustrates precisely the difference between medicine and nursing. The nurse at the bedside is also 'reading the patient' through regular observations, readings, drawing off blood and so on, but the patient remains present. Zussman's representation of medicine 'doing physiology' and nurses 'caring' is a stark but useful analysis. As one of the residents in his study remarked:

> Because a lot of people are intubated, they can't talk. And so you've got to just deal not as a person but as a problem, a set of numbers and dynamics. We're not dealing with a walking talking person. (1992: 36)

In addition to the technical focus of medicine – where there is, the analysis goes, less concern with the personal – Zussman says that the patient disappears in the ICU and reappears as a collection of rights. The culture of rights produces a sense of empowerment for patients and their families and represents one of the main changes in the social context in which health care takes place. Zussman (1992: 97) notes that whilst medicine recognises these rights and thus involves relatives in the broad direction of the management of the patient's care, whether for instance it should be aggressive cure or not, what the physicians are not prepared to do is to allow families to decide about specific treatment interventions. In other words, Zussman's analysis is that the medical profession has conceded the fact that they do not have the power to take the moral decisions about how a patient should be treated; however, by 'reserving some decisions to themselves as matters of technique', medicine retains control. One of the major arguments in Zussman's work is that the physicians appropriate value judgements and then convert them into technical issues and therefore they become part of the province of medicine. This produces a situation in which there is no dispute over the rights of the patient or family representative, but when it comes to decisions about appropriateness of treatments, in other words the technical clinical decisions, medicine remains in control. The difference is between saying 'withdraw or withhold a life-supporting treatment' – a moral decision – and saying that in this case 'it would be futile or in some other way inadvisable, burdensome and so on' – a technical decision. Zussman sums this up by saying:

> The point in question is not whether patients have rights. All agree that they do. Neither is the question whether those rights may be exercised on behalf of the patient by the patient's family. Most agree that they may. Rather, the issue becomes one of the limits of rights, of the boundaries between matters of value and matters of technical knowledge. (1992: 97)

It is worth reiterating here that the United Kingdom position on the role of the family is different. They are consulted when the patient is unable to express a view, but at law the family does not have the final say; that lies with the medical profession, who of course are keen to know what the family view is. However, what Zussman's analysis makes clear is that in the USA the medical profession do retain some of the control of the decisions by virtue of their expertise which the family does not have. So it is then that the medical profession, not the law, defines what constitutes aggressive treatment and when it is appropriate. In this way Zussman says the medical profession can avoid legal issues and retain control of the clinical management of the patient.

Some hospital policies have insisted that medical staff discuss with all patients the possibility of the need for resuscitation arising and their preferred treatment in such an event. Hospital policy can lead to many unnecessary conversations between doctors and patients which create more distress than the supposed benefits that this informed and open approach to care could produce. A well intentioned policy can produce unintended consequences, leading to a situation where it makes better sense for doctors to take a view in advance about their patients – working out who, if they did arrest, could not benefit from resuscitation, and on that premise not raising the question with those patients in the first place.

The combination of the decline in power of medicine and the increase in legal involvement and governmental intervention in health care, along with the rise of nursing's ambitions for independent practice and professionalisation, has altered the social context of professional attitudes and interprofessional disputes. With the move towards multi-professional patient-centred health care where old professional boundaries shift to allow new ways of organising care and sharing the work involved, the future health care workforce will be a rather different entity.

The data from various studies (Anspach 1987; Chambliss 1996; Jennings 1986; 1990; McHaffie and Fowlie 1996; Melia 2001; Seymour 2000; Walby et al. 1994; Zussman 1992) all demonstrate the interprofessional differences of opinion that lead to the production of the rather stereotypical view of nursing and medicine. Mason (personal communication 1999) commented that he had noticed

> an increasing distinction being made between doctoring and nursing in the hospital setting. In the absurd extreme this manifests itself as every doctor being seen as a dangerous paternalist whilst every nurse is regarded as a potential whistle-blower.

As the two main players in health care there is much to be gained from nursing and medicine working together on the basis of a real understanding of each other's roles, rather than falling back on stereotypes which are fast becoming outmoded.

The British Medical Association has always had more to say about nursing than the nursing associations have had to say about medicine. For instance a publication from its Ethics, Science and Information Division, *Medical ethics today*, has around two pages on nursing including this: 'It is clear that doctors and nurses should respect each other's area of expertise and benefit from the particular insights of each' (1993: 288).

LAW AND MEDICINE

On closer examination of the ethnographic data that we have on this matter of interprofessional working practices we find that there is some evidence of an understanding of one another's standpoint (Melia 2001; Seymour 2000). In truth, this is an understanding of the different work that each professional undertakes. The common problem which they both face is the difficulty that comes with decisions which have to be made about patient management: medicine making the decisions and nursing acting upon them. Both professions are responsible for seeing the patient through the consequences of those decisions, and doing so in the context of medical/technological possibilities and societal expectations. There are, and should be, differences between the roles of medicine and of nursing, the former essentially diagnosing and prescribing and the latter providing the support, care and treatment. This, as the data show time and again, will give a different perspective on the patient. Physicians have, as Atkinson (1995) well demonstrates, a focus on the disease, whilst nursing concentrates more on the total patient experience.

It should be remembered that these are matters of focus and emphasis and not mutually exclusive perspectives. It is neither helpful nor true to insist that medicine is about cure and nursing about care and that by extension only nurses are concerned with the patient. This line of argument suggests that medicine does not have a sense of the patient as well as the disease. Medical school curricula have long since taken on board both the social and the medical models: diagnosis and prescription are discussed in the social context of the patients' lives.

All of these factors come together to explain, up to a point, why it is that nurses think that they are the ones close to the patient whilst the medical staff appear to be more remote, doing science and making decisions – decisions which nurses are responsible for carrying through. Nurses are, of course, in the same position with respect to legal judgements. As Zussman (1992) and others have noted, the patient is increasingly taking the role of litigant. When court orders are sought resulting in the continuation or withdrawal of treatment, it is the nurse who has the more sustained contact with the patient whilst the legal decisions are carried through.

Some of the disputes between nursing and medicine do arise from this question of nurses being saddled with medicine's decisions. Nursing has to recognise that for all the custom and practice of a joint approach, in the end a medical decision has to be taken. Medicine, for its part, has to recognise the consequences of its decisions for other health care professionals. In the UK the most important case in legal terms is that of Anthony Bland who was crushed in a football stadium disaster in April 1989. For a long while he was deprived of oxygen and his cerebral cortex was destroyed; however his brain still functioned so he had a heartbeat and breathed by himself. Airedale NHS Trust went to court to request legal sanction to remove the nutrition and hydration from a patient in a persistent vegetative state. He was in the PVS until March 1993 when, after a House of Lords ruling, permission was given to withdraw tube-feeding and he died nine days later. This decision had the full support of the family and hospital staff.[1]

The Bland case attracted a lot of media attention and produced a long debate in medicine and nursing, with strong arguments being mounted on both sides of the question of whether tube-feeding is a medical treatment. During the course of Anthony Bland's illness the BMA had been asked to produce guidelines for the treatment of people in PVS. A committee took evidence and studied the literature but failed to come up with guidance. Their problem lay in part in the fact that the law was not very clear about withdrawal of treatment.

The Bland case went first to the High Court: the neurologist and family sought a declaration that to stop feeding him by tube would not be unlawful. (It would not have been unlawful under Scots law.) The High Court ruling in November 1992 was that 'his spirit had left him and all that remains is the shell of his body'. The wording was that Airedale NHS Trust and the responsible physician

> may lawfully discontinue all life-sustaining treatment and medical support measures designed to keep Anthony Bland alive in his existing persistent vegetative state, including the termination of ventilation, nutrition and hydration by artificial means, and they may lawfully discontinue and thereafter need not furnish medical treatment to him except for the sole purpose of enabling Anthony Bland to end his life and die peacefully with the greatest dignity and with the least distress.

There is often thought to be a technological drive in medical treatment, 'if we can do it, we should' – rather like the reason we climb mountains, 'because they are there'. The Bland case is not so much (to continue the metaphor) a mountain too far, but rather one that Anthony Bland and his doctors got stranded upon. The burden of Anthony Bland's plight fell on his family, and the nursing and medical staff of the hospital. By all accounts they worked well together as a team and the NHS Trust laid on professional counselling as well as peer support, which was important for the survival of the health care professionals. The consultant in charge said that, in the four years Anthony Bland was cared for, only one nurse felt that she could not go with the decision (personal communication).

Nurses frequently make the case that they are the patient's advocates. This, as I have argued in Chapter 1, is not a helpful stance as it works against teamwork and at times the duty of care. The 'advocate' is a legal concept: it has no useful place in the nurse–patient relationship and even less in the context of health care teamwork. One extension of this argument is to regard nursing as some kind of watchdog for medical practice. Appalling though this idea is, it comes through in some of the discussions of nursing ethics, usually in the context of 'nurse as patient advocate' discussions.

The idea that nurses should provide some kind of brake on medical practice is neither desirable nor practical. Notwithstanding the widely held view on nursing and advocacy, it seems to me that nurses should not attempt to play gatekeeper to medicine's advances. Teamworking and appropriate division of labour are preferable.

The boundaries between care, cure and palliation, as we have said, shade into each other. The decision to adopt one or the other approach is not a clear-cut one. The social context of health care and the power relationship between the professions are important here. As noted above, this rather well trodden path of the power of the professions misses some of the finer points of interprofessional working practices. However, the interprofessional boundaries are social constructions, just as are the boundaries between ethical and technical judgements, as Zussman points out. He is talking about technical decisions being taken with no reference being made to the family. When this happens he describes it in terms of 'ethics is transformed into medicine' (1992: 151). We are not looking at an either/or here: the clinical and technical decisions have to be taken and acted upon in a social context. The technical decisions are problematic, the ways in which they are arrived at are social processes (McHaffie and Fowlie 1996; Melia 2001; Seymour 2000) and they involve social and organisational aspects of care and practice.

The balance between the three sides of the care–cure–palliation triangle is also in many ways a social construction. Medicine, by virtue of taking the clinical decisions, tends to harden the stereotype of medicine pursuing the technical part of the work; this in turn leaves open the way for nurses not only to lay claim to the holistic caring aspect of health care work, but also to lay claim to the role of patient's advocate. This is in essence the old debate about care and cure; it is something of a straw man, and its proponents are usually those attempting to stake a claim to a particular role for nursing. This can easily be done without making the case that medical work is somehow uncaring by virtue of its focus on the diagnostic and the technical aspects of medicine.

Seymour discusses the difficulties in moving a patient out of ICU once intensive care is no longer appropriate and the patient is dying. She notes that on the basis of her data 'the issue of continuity of care across the health care system is revealed as problematic' (2000: 161). We can see here how the social context and the labels we recognise in the social world come sharply into focus in the clinical reality of effecting health care. The ways in which we frame care and the ways in which it is delivered have implications for the decisions made and the working practices. The context of care is made clear in the point raised by Seymour. Once a patient has been moved out of the ICU on grounds of the futility of continuing with aggressive treatment, the standards against which his progress is measured change. Survival is no longer an expectation. The labels of 'intensive care' and 'terminal care' carry a whole set of expectations and ethical assumptions about the nature and style of care that the patients will receive.

As we have noted, debates and disagreements which take place between nursing and medicine are often characterised in terms of nurses adopting the 'caring' rhetoric and awarding the role of 'curer' or sometimes 'failed curer' to medicine. As we said in Chapter 1, nursing has certainly paid a good deal of attention to the ethic of care, not least as this was part of nursing's project to achieve its goal of professional status. The literature in the caring ethics field usually presents a rather rigid, probably false and certainly disingenuous dichotomy, with medicine being about diagnosis and cure and nursing being about care. This line of argument does not take us very far. There is a long tradition of adopting a power analysis approach to the relationship between medicine and nursing (Freidson 1970; 1994; Mackay 1993; Witz 1992). This approach fits with the finding that consensus is all-important for effective teamworking in ICU; the point is that there is a hierarchy of professions which could be the operational basis of an ICU, but this would not produce good teamwork and care. For the same reasons there is a need for flexibility in approach to the care–cure–palliation triangle.

The difficulties in deciding how to approach the triangle are perhaps less about professional turf-based disputes, notably between nursing and medicine, and more about the problem of getting the balance right between societal expectations and clinical and technical possibilities. The power relationship between the professions of nursing and medicine is not to be discounted, as it is very much a part of the social context of health care and the organisation of clinical practice is not unaffected by these relationships (Walby et al. 1994).

We may be some good way off the notion of a health care professional with less focus on the old disciplinary boundaries. However, this may be a good juncture at which to develop ground rules for ethics in health care which have less to do with professional concerns and more to do with the ethical dimension of a patient-led service. I have characterised this as health care ethics in order to emphasise the move away from the parallel existence of medical ethics and nursing ethics.

As the issues are complex and centre upon the quality of life, there is clearly a case for placing the patient at the centre of the ethical debate. One of the purposes of this book is to make the case for health care ethics, as opposed to medical ethics or nursing ethics, and perhaps even more generally to make the case for conceiving of health caring as a professional activity undertaken by a professional group of health care workers. Health caring is then effected by a team of health care professionals, albeit a heterogeneous group made up of the different disciplines concerned with health, working together, drawing upon different knowledge bases for the specialist areas of the work – diagnosis, treatment, care, therapy and so on. What this team would have in common is the role of a professional in health care. This group of health carers then stands in need of ground rules for health caring – rules which would in many ways of course resemble the ethical codes that currently exist in the different disciplines in health care. The difference would lie in the move away from the profession-centred approach to ethics to a more patient-focused one.

As we have seen, the extent to which the law is involved in health care is increasing. Zussman (1992) argues that there has been a shift towards patients' rights and legal rulings and away from medical dominance. The ethical issues which developments and advances in medical science bring often require legal clarity to be brought to clinical decisions. However that may be, there is still a place for clinical judgement which is informed by ethical reflection. This judgement, it should be remembered, takes place in a social context which is every bit as important in the shaping of that judgement, as is the law and the current state of medical science.

CLINICAL JUDGEMENT AND THE TECHNOLOGICAL IMPERATIVE

We tend to think of clinical judgements as medical judgements. However, given what we have noted about the complex nature of the interaction between technology and the social context of human communication and emotion in health care, there is a place for thinking about nursing judgement. This position has been neatly summed up by Seymour in her concluding discussion of withholding medical treatment in ICU:

> Focusing on the intricacies of social interaction in the specialised environment of intensive care helps to shed light on the way in which the paradox of 'natural' and 'artificial' is dealt with at the bedside and how the disparate understandings of medical science and clinical wisdom are reconciled. (2000: 104)

This notion of clinical wisdom is, I think, especially useful, as it captures that area where clinical judgement, clinical chemistry and ethical concerns intersect. Clinical wisdom is also something which is difficult both to define and to learn. If health care becomes too fenced about by legal precedent, technical predictions and overly standardised practices (the downside of evidence-based medicine), it is clinical wisdom that will disappear through the back door whilst we are looking the other way, preoccupied with setting benchmarks, gold standards and guidelines for practice.

The idea of judgement in health care is of course not new, as we noted in Chapter 1. Aristotle spoke of 'practical wisdom' as one of the virtues required to produce a moral agent who is skilled and has integrity. In the clinical situation, health care professionals, nursing and medical, need a combination of technical and scientific competence balanced by the moral dimension, the wisdom to arrive at practice which will be in the interests of patients.

The care–cure–palliation triangle offers a means of thinking about the consequences of following the technological imperative when it comes to high-technology-driven medicine. In the ICU we have seen that there is a tendency to err on the side of caution and probably to over-admit as a result. Jennings notes that 'the prevailing moral calculus is to err on the side of over-treating some so that the moral risk of under-treating any will be minimised' (1990: 224).

Caution can lead to difficult decisions about withdrawal of treatment. The lessons drawn here from intensive care can be translated to oncology and palliative care where we find similar ethical dilemmas when aggressive anti-cancer treatments have been tried and failed. The same question prevails: when is it reasonable to call a halt, or indeed when is it reasonable to go on? The balance of doing harm and doing good, the respect for autonomy, and at a wider level the questions of resources, are relevant in this field of care.

In the last chapter we looked at the proper use of the ICU; in this chapter the focus has moved a little, towards the proper use of treatment. An understanding of when it is acceptable, morally right, to move to the care side of the triangle and prepare for death then becomes the expectation and goal. In many cases this move is self-evident and there is no real problem with the management of the final stages of care. But in a social setting which has become very technologically driven, and where there is a generalised death defying ethos, calling a halt, even when it is clinically and morally the right thing to do, is not always that simple.

The social context and the ways of working in the different sectors of health care play a part in structuring the kinds of decisions which are made about treatment. The discussion in this chapter has been about the differences and similarities in care, cure and palliative approaches to the management of patient care. The tendency towards cure and the expectations of society have brought us to a position where the ICU is a routine part of the provision in a developed health care service. I have argued in Chapter 2 that the existence of intensive care shapes practice in other areas. In this chapter the discussion has moved beyond the ICU, but the influence of intensive care and the parallel high tech approaches adopted in oncology raise similar ethical issues.

The consideration of the care–cure–palliation triangle brings some of the issues into focus. It should be not so much the care–cure debate that exercises professionals in health care but rather the question of where technology leads and how society's urge to stave off death shapes health care thinking and practice. It cannot be the case that a 'life at any cost' approach to disease will result in the best interests of patients being served. In the end what is required is a balance, a judgement and a focus on the patient. We need to avoid technological imperatives where they are not sensible and to recognise that the law does not always provide the solution, as we have seen in the limitations of advance directives.

Boyd's conclusion makes a fitting close to this chapter:

> while a living will may make it less likely that someone's terminal suffering is prolonged by modern medical technology, it can never replace the current role of the scientific and humane clinical judgement of the doctors and nurses into whose care the patient is delivered. (1999: 7)

NOTES

1   *Airedale NHS Trust* v. *Bland* [1993] 1 All ER 821.

iv caring for bodies, caring for people

SOCIOLOGY OF THE BODY

One of the frequent reminders offered to health care professionals is that 'patients are people'. This is not because health care staff do not know this or, worse, do not care about the status of their patients. It is simply that in the cut and thrust of decision making in relation to the clinical management of a patient's condition, the human side of health care can be overshadowed by its technical aspects.

Cartesian ideas about a mind-body dichotomy took philosophers down the binary route to understanding human existence, and for some while this was the dominant mode of thinking. The body–person duality of the individual presents a problem for clinicians and, in theoretical terms, the same duality has exercised philosophers and presents a problem for sociologists. This duality is expressed rather differently by sociologists, moral philosophers and clinicians. These differences are explored in this chapter. In clinical situations the body sometimes carries the two meanings together, that is to say the 'body' that is being cared for is also someone's relative, friend and so on, and health care staff can imagine the 'person'; this makes the work hard and emotionally charged. In this chapter we explore the dilemmas which these different versions of the body present for clinicians, patients and their families and consider the sociological perspectives on the body.

It is often said that sociology came late to the body. Turner's (1992) explanation of sociology's lack of focus on the body is that sociology followed philosophy, especially Descartes, in accepting a mind–body dichotomy and so went on to focus on the mind as the entity which defines that which we recognise as human. Turner (1984; 1987; 1991; 1995) is one of the main protagonists of the sociology of the body. He notes that whilst social anthropology saw the importance of the body, sociology did not. In his introduction to a discussion of the recent devel-

opments in the theory of the body, Turner recognises that the work of
Erving Goffman 'was significant in alerting social theorists to the role of
the body in the construction of a social person' (1991: 11). Turner's complaint, however, is that Goffman never produced 'a specific theory of
embodiment'. For Turner, sociology's interest in the body should be
about how social practices transform the human body. In the preface of
his work *Regulating bodies*, Turner says:

> the history of the West was not so much the transformation of cul-
> ture under the impact of rationality as the transformation of the
> human body via a myriad of practices. Medicalisation, secularisa-
> tion and rationalisation appeared to be the great forces which had
> operated on the body, or more properly on the body-in-the-every-
> day-world. (1992: 4)

Turner argues that with the exception of G.H. Mead, Goffman and
Bourdieu,

> there appears to be a rationalistic bias in sociology which has until
> recently treated the social actor as a disembodied rational agent
> ... from Weber onwards, the body appears in sociological theory
> as a feature of the environment. (1992: 23)

Given the volume of Goffman's work and the importance of his contribution, it is difficult to sidestep it as lightly as Turner appears to in
staking his own claim to being a central mover in the sociology of the
body project. Not that Mead or Goffman claimed to be producing theories of the body; it may be that they did not see the need rather than it
being an oversight on their part. It is worth noting that Turner is paint-
ing on a wider canvas, for although he is writing in the subspeciality of
medical sociology, or more properly the sociology of health and illness,[1]
he sees the sociology of the body as a link back into mainstream sociology. He notes that there are worries around in medical sociology that
'The leading figures of medical sociology today appear to make few contributions to the development of sociology as such' (1992: 24). This is in
contrast to leading figures of the past – Parsons (1951), Roth (1963),
Glaser and Strauss (1967) – whose work in medical sociology also contributed to the thinking and concerns of mainstream sociology.

In 1992 Turner elaborated upon the ideas first propounded in his
book *Medical power and social knowledge* (1987) when he suggested that
the solution to the gap between the subspeciality and sociology would
be to 'develop a sociology of the body as a theoretical programme in
medical sociology as a bridge with theoretical sociology' (1992: 24). By
1995 Turner was saying that, following a stream of major work on the
body, there was still a lack of a coherent theory of the body:

> Although it is no longer possible to believe that the question of

the body has been neglected, as yet we do not possess a coherent and comprehensive theory of the body which would address
the problems related to human embodiment, the body and body
image. My argument is that a sociologically adequate medical
sociology is dependent upon the creation of a coherent sociology
of the body. (1995: 229)

I, for my part, had embarked on this book thinking that the sociology of
the body literature might have something to offer those interested in ethical issues involved in caring for bodies. I set out with a dose of scepti-
cism as I find some of the arguments in the sociology of the body writings rather circular and ultimately not very helpful. The argument seems
to be that it is the body's consciousness of itself that is important. My
problem here is that the body's consciousness of itself sounds more like
the mind than the body. More fundamentally, the theory of the body literature often appears to be little more than semantics. The word 'corporeality' is frequently used to stress the meaning of the body, but this really takes us no further with the question of the utility of a theory of the
body, as corporeality means relating to the physical material body as
opposed to the spiritual self. So, a body is a body, then what, or even so
what? An example of this near tautology comes in Frank's analytic
review of the sociology of the body literature, when he says:

To think of 'society' having a social order problem is more tyranny of the abstract. Bodies certainly have problems among other
bodies, but the point is to hold on to the fundamental embodiment of these problems rather than allowing the problems to be
abstracted from the needs, pains and desires of bodies. (1991: 91)

To be sure, the point that Frank makes goes beyond a simple statement
that social actors have physical bodies, but the abstractions which he
objects to are the means by which we discuss needs, pain and so on.

Shilling (1993) talks about the body as 'something of an absent presence in sociology'. As he puts it:

It is our bodies which allow us to act, to intervene in and to alter
the flow of daily life. Indeed it is impossible to have an adequate
theory of human agency without taking into account the body. In
a very important sense, acting people are acting bodies. (1993: 9)

Again, I may be missing something but this does seem to be a statement
of the obvious. It is interesting to note in passing that whilst Shilling and
others are critical of classical sociology for having left the body out of
social theory, it is the human body that functionalists used as the analogy for the description of self-regulating social systems (Comte,
Durkheim, Parsons). The ideas of balance and equilibrium are very
much the stuff of bodies.

In the 1990s sociology became interested in the sociology of the body.[2] Frank notes in an analytic review of the sociology ot the body literature that:

> The sociology of the body argues for the re-conceptualisation of social theory. The grounding of theory must be the body's consciousness of itself ... Only on this grounding can theory put selves into bodies and bodies into society. (1991: 91)

Again, this does not sound to me too far removed from a concern with the mind or at least the intellectual aspect of the person. Despite the Cartesian split between mind and body, medicine has taken a good deal of interest in the interplay between mind and body in the disease process and the process of recovery.

Frank also examines the case for a sociology of the body and how this might inform what he and others (Feher 1989) term 'an ethics of the body'. Frank concludes that:

> Ultimately there would be no ethics of the body, rather all ethics would take the body as its fundamental point of departure. Thus also there would be no sociology of the body, but rather fundamental embodiment of social action would ground all sociology. (1991: 85)

Frank says that the reason for this is simple: it is that

> only bodies suffer. Only by a studied concentration on the body can we bear adequate witness to this suffering. Only an ethics or a social science which witnesses suffering is worthy of our energies or attention. (1991: 95–6)

Shilling's (1993) work on the body and social theory includes a discussion of a range of Giddens's work, including that on self-identity and high modernity (Giddens 1991). Shilling says that the body is now so central to a sense of identity that death assumes more significance for people than it has at other times in our history. I would suggest that it is not so much the centrality of the body to our identity that makes death so significant; it is rather that we have as a society come to depend upon medicine to find ways to delay death – and some might urge to prevent it altogether.

Shilling also notes that Giddens's (1979; 1984) commentary on the body complements his ideas on the relationship between structure and agency, in so far as 'Human bodies are themselves the medium and the outcome of human (reproductive) labour product' (1993: 201). Bodies, he goes on, both constrain action and allow intervention in everyday life. Shilling's complaint about Giddens's position is that Giddens with his structuration theory does not 'specify how we go about ascertaining conditions under which bodies constrain and enable action' (1993: 201). As Shilling puts it, 'Giddens's writings alternate between presenting us with voluntaristic and deterministic views of the body' (1993: 201). This complaint is rather obscure, and it is not easy, it has to be said, to see what such a separation of constraint and enabling would look like if it were elaborated.

Giddens (1991) has a refreshingly straightforward view on this question of body: he says 'The self, of course, is embodied' (1991: 56). He goes on, 'The body is not simply an entity, but is experienced as a practical mode of coping with external situations and events' (1991: 56).

Shilling says that the tendency for sociology to focus on the mind meant that 'the body was usually considered as a passive container which acted as a shell to the active mind (which was identified with distinguishing humans from animals)' (1993: 26). Shilling states at several points in his book that sociology as a discipline has rarely focused on the body as an area of investigation in its own right; yet, he goes on to say, sociology has had to deal with aspects of human embodiment. This does not seem to be all that surprising. In the discourse of health care ethics and medical sociology, where bodies come with the territory, it is perhaps the case that bodies in their own right do get overlooked, as do the taken-for-granteds in other areas of life. It seems to be not much more than semantic niceties to debate the embodiment aspects of social life, because it is the case that social life and social action require bodies.

Strauss et al. in *The social organisation of medical work* note one issue that arose from their observation of medical work:

An obvious feature of this work is that patients' bodies are central to that work – central in the sense that bodies are malfunctioning and must be helped or at least managed, central also insofar as things are done to or with bodies or their parts or systems. (1985: 260)

THE BODY AND DEATH

The split of mind from body is not perhaps so much the problem for health care professionals; rather it is the separation of the physical body from the notion of personhood. It is the body as ethical territory, perhaps, that is of interest. There are plainly times in an emergency situation – a frequent occurrence in an ICU but it happens elsewhere too – when the needs of the physical body have to come first. However, there is always the person to consider as well. There are rights to be respected, needs to be met and a general recognition that it is a life that is being cared for and treated, not simply a body. The interdependence of the two – life and body – is clear, especially when the body's pathology threatens the life contained in that body or threatens its quality.

The writings of moral philosophers and lawyers take the discussion of dilemmas relating to the caring for bodies further than does the sociology of the body literature. Intensive care, as we have said, provides the occasion for ethical debate when clinical cases and situations present in a singularly dramatic way. Caring for people who are being ventilated, especially when they are unconscious, sharpens up our perspective on the human body and its relationship to the person. The meaning that the body carries when it is in a fully autonomous conscious state is different from that carried by a body in an unconscious state. The latter more obviously signals a very clear need for assistance. Also, as we are aware of the usual condition of the body, that is a body in the fully autonomous charge of its owner, the unconscious body makes us aware of the need to protect the rights of that person as these cannot be asserted or claimed in the usual way. The body in persistent vegetative state (PVS), and the body being perfused and ventilated prior to donating organs for transplantation to another person, present very similar concerns for nursing in that they are bodies rather than persons.

The persistent vegetative state is a

> clinical condition of complete unawareness of the self and the environment, accompanied by sleep–wake cycles with either complete or partial preservation of hypothalamic and brainstem autonomic functions. (Task Force 1994)

Patients in PVS also show no evidence that they are capable of sustained purposeful responses to stimuli.

There are two routes to the tissue anoxia which, when permanent, constitutes death. These are respiratory failure and cardiac failure. In either case the diagnostic problem lies in the definition of permanence (Mason and McCall Smith 1999). Respiration and circulation can be restored and assisted artificially. For both to function they are dependent on the brainstem; when this fails – brain death – a person can be pronounced dead.

The two major catastrophes for the brain are brain death and PVS. It was Jennett who first published on the problems of PVS in a paper in the *Lancet* subtitled 'a syndrome in search of a name' (Jennett and Plum 1972). Since that time there has been much debate and public discussion of this complex medical problem and on more than one occasion the law has been consulted for clarification of what the proper action should be. Jennett puts the problem clearly when he says:

> Patients with irrecoverable severe brain damage may be brain dead or in a persistent vegetative state (PVS). In the former it is the brainstem which is irreversibly out of action, in the latter the cerebral cortex. These result in two contrasting physiological situations and two quite different problems for decision making. In

brain death, the paradox is a patient whose brain is no longer
functioning but whose heart continues to beat. In the vegetative
state, the paradox is of a patient who is awake but is not aware.
(1996: 13)

The brain dead patient will only survive for a week or so even with full
life support. By contrast those in PVS, where breathing is spontaneous,
provided that they are tube-fed and given basic care, may survive for
many years: this is the tragedy of their condition and the reason that the
law is brought into the clinical decision making process.

The distinction between life and death or, more properly, between
being alive and being dead, is not so straightforward as was once the
case. When the possibility of resuscitation of a person whose cardiac and
respiratory activity had ceased arrived on the scene, 'dead' became a
complicated category. With the arrival of resuscitation the traditional
way of declaring that someone was dead was thrown into question. The
possibility of organ transplantation brought with it a second reason for
rethinking the definition of 'dead'.

Prior to the 1950s and before the advent of resuscitation, the evidence of death was the absence of a pulse and the cessation of breathing.
The arrival of these two symptoms signalled death. Now those same
indicators may be a trigger for resuscitation. It will not always be clinically or morally appropriate to resuscitate depending on the length of
time that the brain has lacked oxygen, but the possibility of resuscitation
exists and this has had a profound effect on clinical medicine.

Jones states the problem neatly when he says:

the technological ability to sustain brain dead patients whose bodies are biologically living has made it necessary to determine
whether the continued provision of health care for such patients
serves any useful purpose, and whether organs from such bodies
could be used for transplantation purposes. (2000: 198)

Jones goes on, drawing on Engelhardt's paper 'Re-examining the definition of death and becoming clearer about what it is to be alive' (1988), to
say: 'In other words, is transplantation a matter of stealing organs from
living persons or salvaging organs from the still-living bodies of the
dead?' (2000: 198).

These two advances in modern medicine – resuscitation and transplantation – made it necessary to develop a precise way of determining
when someone was indeed dead, and the concept of brain death
emerged. Two neuro-physicians, Mollaret and Goulon (1959), were the
first to describe what is now known as 'brain death'; they called it *le coma
depassé*, which translates literally to 'a state beyond coma'. The widely
accepted definition of brain death came out of the Harvard Medical
School (1968). There followed what Jones (2000: 200) called 'intensive

debate' in many countries about the relationship between 'brain death' and 'death'. As medicine became more knowledgeable about brain death, the importance of the brainstem was recognised. The brainstem is the site of the respiratory centre and when it fails, usually as a result of pressure in the brain, the clinical signs of bodily death are apparent.

The notion of brain death put into question the status of more traditional definitions of death. The question was whether a patient who was brain dead was indeed dead; this was an especially crucial question when there was no stopping of the heart. Transplant surgeons were especially anxious to have this matter clear. The Conference of Medical Royal Colleges and their Faculties in the UK produced two reports. The first, 'Diagnosis of brain death' (1976), stated that 'permanent functional death of the brainstem constitutes brain death and that once this has occurred further artificial support is fruitless and should be withdrawn'. Skegg notes that 'the report did not express any view on whether such patients could be regarded as dead before artificial ventilation was withdrawn and cardiac arrest occurred' (1988: 192). This he suggests was in order to gain agreement to the extent that was achieved by the Conference; any more would have been too far for the state of thinking at the time.

Whilst the definition of brain death clearly pointed the way for the patient in question, it did not help the transplant team. The second report by the Conference of Medical Royal Colleges and their Faculties in the UK, 'Diagnosis of death' (1979), established that once brain death had occurred 'a person was dead, even though heartbeat continued'. This report did, as Skegg puts it, 'what many had wrongly assumed that the earlier report had done. It accepted the view that whatever the mode of its production, brain death represents the stage at which a patient becomes truly dead' (1988: 194). The 'Diagnosis of death' report concludes that:

> the identification of brain death means that the patient is dead, whether or not the function of some organs, such as a heartbeat, is still maintained by artificial means. (1979: para. 9)

The statement makes the position clear for the transplant service and paved the way for both beating-heart donors and elective ventilation of patients who have been declared brain dead but who were not intensive care patients on ventilators. Lamb (1996) notes that the definition of brain death in addition to death is confusing. He says: 'either the patient is dead or he is not, in an absolute sense. Being brain dead can suggest a special way of being dead, which like "virtually dead" is misleading' (1996: 18). The point Lamb makes is an important one and highlights the fact that this is not a new way of death, it is simply a new definition which medical technological advances have necessitated. It is interesting to note in passing that Skegg (1988: 192) says that by 1978 there were more than thirty published sets of criteria for brain death.

This clarity about the definition of death is important. In connection with the question of when does dead mean dead, another publication of 1979 was the Department of Health and Social Security's code of practice for the removal of organs from cadavers (DHSS 1979). This code has it that death can be determined by 'the irreversible cessation of brainstem function – brain death'. Jones (2000) points out that the importance of this definition was that it established the position that once brain death occurs a person is dead despite the fact of a continuing heartbeat. As he puts it: 'this expresses the viewpoint that brain dead individuals are no longer living human beings' (2000: 201).

The consequences of these definitions and the practices which lead from them – that is the decision not to continue with life support and the possibility of organ donation – are not without problems. Returning to a point touched upon earlier, it is the case that from the nursing viewpoint the needs of a body are much the same whatever the situation. Whether an individual is in persistent vegetative state, or undergoing elective ventilation and perfusion with fluids prior to becoming a beating-heart donor, they exist in the form of a body – a body which demands respect by virtue of the life it contained. In a more general sense it is expected that in a civilised society the human body, dead or alive, is treated with respect. The status of the two bodies, the one in PVS and the other a donor cadaver, is quite different in human and one might reasonably say emotional terms.

The kinds of distinctions that we are beginning to see coming from these attempts to be clear about definitions of death are made in terms of physiology and some other human, emotional quality of living. As Jones says, decisions about the state of a brain dead person 'cannot avoid for long reference to "personal life" and "bodily life"' (2000: 202). Skegg says:

> When a patient is brain dead but his or her body is maintained on an artificial ventilator, the cardiovascular, gastrointestinal and urinary systems continue to function. The body is warm, consumes oxygen and may react to harmful stimuli. It would be difficult to describe this as a 'dead body'. (1988: 206)

NOT DEAD, NOT DYING

This situation of a person being 'brain dead' yet 'biologically alive' is unsettling and, notwithstanding clear clinical and legal positions, remains rather confusing for those caring for them. However, Jones, following Skegg (1988), has pointed out that whilst it might be hard to think of a brain dead ventilated body as a dead body, the alternatives are equally awkward. Jones states: 'Any disadvantages in viewing a brain dead person as dead have to be weighed against the disadvantage of regarding a brain dead patient as a "ventilated corpse" or a "beating-heart cadaver"' (2000: 202).

The idea that brain death and persistent vegetative state are related – both at some kind of halfway stage between life and death – is not only misleading but wrong. Lamb puts the position very sharply when he says:

> when terms like 'brain death' and 'vegetative state' are used as if they were synonymous (in proposals for euthanasia or termination of treatment) there is not only factual error but serious risk of ethical abuse. Patients in a vegetative state are not dead. No culture in the world would consider them as fit for burial, organ removal, experimentation etc. (1996: 6)

As we have noted, the nursing requirements of a person in PVS are not dissimilar to those of an unconscious patient or a beating-heart cadaver. This is why the PVS is of such clinical and ethical interest. The vegetative state puts patients into a no man's land: as Wikler (1988) puts it, 'not dead, not dying'. Patients in PVS do not have a terminal condition but they are dependent for their continued existence upon medical support and nursing care. As Wikler says, the life they endure can be described as 'the lowest functioning phase of life or the highest functioning phase of death' (1988: 42).

Again it is the social practices in ICU which reveal a good deal as well as the moral debates. Managing emotions and remaining optimistic is a demanding part of the work. We should remember too that in the clinical setting these patients are among others with rather better prognoses. One of the most difficult things for health care workers to bring off is the change of approach and mood when they move between the relatives of the brain dead patients and those of the more hopeful cases.

The consequences of PVS can be far reaching. For example the British Medical Association (1994) guidelines on treatment decisions for patients in PVS say that no decision should be taken to withdraw in the first twelve months. Thus, they say, 'the question of whether it is morally appropriate to keep a pregnant woman alive for the sake of her foetus alone does not arise' (1994: 4). The question of pregnancy and brain death is for another day, but in the context of this work it is interesting to note how this BMA guidance converts the moral issue into a technical one and so avoids the difficulty. I would not judge the view to be right or wrong, but simply note the ingenuity of bypassing a tricky moral issue by the simple means of setting a time frame. Ironically, it is the stability of the PVS which makes it so problematic. In medical parlance, 'stable' is usually good news, or at least not bad news. Here it is neither: it is stuck in a state of not living and not dying. Jones makes a very sensitive comment on the situation where there is brain death yet the body 'lives' on:

> The apparent life of the patient's body should be handled sensi-
> tively, both for relatives and hospital staff, and out of respect for
> the person who was. The living body of a dead patient represents
> the remnants of a human life. (2000: 225)

The now very familiar cases of Karen Quinlan in the United States
and Anthony Bland in England (see Chapter 3) are frequently cited
when PVS and its attendant dilemmas are debated.[3] Lord Justice
Hoffman's description of Anthony Bland's plight is clear:[4]

> His stiffened joints have caused his limbs to be rigidly contracted so
> that his arms are tightly flexed across his chest and his legs unnaturally
> contorted. Reflex movements in the throat cause him to vomit and dribble.
> Of all this and the presence of members of his family who take turns to visit
> him, Anthony Bland has no consciousness at all. The parts of his brain
> which provided him with consciousness have turned to fluid.[5]

Karen Quinlan when aged 21 had a cardiac arrest following an acciden-
tal overdose of prescription sedatives and alcohol. She was in what now
would be termed PVS: indeed it was her case which propelled the condition into the ethical limelight. She was placed on a ventilator but when
it became clear that she would not recover her parents asked that her
ventilator be switched off. It was a surprise to all concerned that she
went on to live nine more years in PVS. The Quinlans' lawyers claimed
that the respirator constituted 'extraordinary means' of keeping her
alive: the doctors disputed this and so the case went to court. The
Supreme Court allowed the discontinuation of ventilation but made it
clear that this was not about the right to assist suicide.

In relation to the Bland case, Singer notes:

> In making the decision that, for Anthony Bland, continued life
> brought no benefit, and that it can be lawful intentionally to cause
> the death of an innocent human being, the British [sic] courts
> were breaking with the traditional principle of the sanctity of
> human life. (1994: 73)

One of the features of the legal proceedings in similar cases which have
followed is that they can be drawn out as the case is taken to a higher
court if the first request was rejected. The striking thing about the
Quinlan and Bland cases, and others like them, is that by the time the
legal process is complete the patient has been kept alive for years rather
than months. Nancy Cruzan was another American case where the permission of the court had to be sought to withdraw artificial nutrition and
hydration in order to allow her to die rather than continue in PVS. The
strain on all concerned is summed up, and the time frame underscored,

in her tombstone engraving, which Singer reproduced in his book *Rethinking life and death* (1994: 62):

> Nancy Beth Cruzan
> Most loved
> Daughter sister aunt
> Born July 20 1957
> Departed January 11 1983
> At peace December 26 1990

As this makes clear, and Singer notes, 'by this time (1990) she had been supported for nearly eight years and, for at least several of them, it had been clear that she would never regain consciousness' (1994: 62). The time between departing and being at peace represents nearly eight years during which her 'body' was nursed. Only those who have been involved can really have any idea of what that is like. The routines of nursing care and the amazing adaptability of human beings are the two main explanations of how care staff and relatives get through this experience.

Gillett notes that the brain is central to personality and so to life: 'If his brain is no longer working and has no prospect of returning to an adequate level to support this activity, then his liberty as an embodied person has been destroyed' (1986: 84). Gillett's take on the person and the body is one frequently encountered in the ICU. As we have seen, decisions to withdraw treatment are agonisingly difficult to make, but the knowledge of what it is like to care for a brain dead patient puts the decision into perspective. This is one of the genuine dilemmas of health care: that is, whichever course of action is adopted some ethical principle is breached. The cases which have gone to law, Quinlan and Bland, have done so to release both patient and carers from an impossible situation.

Bodies in other circumstances, where the outlook is more hopeful, are still cared for by nurses, but the task is vested with a quite different significance. The prospect of transplant makes the future life of some patients very attractive. ICU staff are of course well aware of the other side of the matter. In practice a large proportion of transplants involve what are termed 'cadaver donated organs' – those coming from patients who after a period of being ventilated in ICU are pronounced brain dead. Mason and McCall Smith say that: 'There is no logical reason why ventilation should not be continued after death and the heart be maintained during an operation for organ donation.' This way, they say, 'The ideal situation of the living donor is achieved in a cadaver' (1999: 351).

This is of course both legal and logical, but as is so often the case the emotions cannot be underestimated in these high tech situations in the ICU. However, on a more objective note, the use of resources has also to be taken into consideration in the context of elective ventilation of beating-heart cadavers. ICU beds which are devoted to the work of the transplant service are not available for more conventional intensive care patients. This represents a problem of resource allocation and an area where fine judgements have to be made.

ENDING LIFE

As we have seen, bodies possess characteristics which would cause us to categorise them as bodies even though they differ functionally. It is arguable as to whether they also differ in moral terms. An immediate response to this might well be that they are not morally distinct entities, because a consequence of arguing along such lines would lead to differing treatment of these bodies in ways which would go against the instincts of the health care professionals. The moral distinctions between the different kinds of bodies described – unconscious ventilated patient, coma patient, elective ventilated brain dead donor and patient in PVS – can be seen at some level. For instance, the use of organs is not acceptable in all societies where for various cultural and religious reasons any violation of the body after death is not allowed. Mason and McCall Smith say that in some countries 'notably in Japan there is an inherent antipathy to the concept of brain death' (1999: 352). They note that this view extends to a large extent to the medical profession, but state however that: 'A Japanese doctor has, in fact, been charged with murder for performing cardiac transplant; although the case was dropped, it did nothing to encourage the evolution of a programme' (1999: 352). The Japanese position (Nudeshima 1991) points to the fact that we cannot equate technical advancement with a moral sophistication in the same direction. It shows the strength of cultural norms and customs and demonstrates how moral stances have roots other than in science and technology.

A perfused and ventilated yet brain dead body is, on the face of it, being shown less respect than one would usually expect a civilised society to show its dead. It is difficult not to embark upon a wedge (as in 'thin end of') argument and see the harvesting of organs as a potential problem here. Horror tales of the markets for organs linked to the push for changes in the law to allow euthanasia, which come up every so often, do not really further this debate. Those in the end stages of motor neurone disease have come into the public eye recently when they have sought to end their lives and required the assistance of others.

Making distinctions between cases which it could be argued are similar is one of the difficult aspects of the intersection of law and ethics. We may feel intuitively that if we are willing to do such and such in case X then the same should be so in case Y. Caring for individuals whose needs appear to be the same but where the legal position is different is a difficult matter.

Two high profile cases which went through the English courts had differing outcomes. Diane Pretty suffered from motor neurone disease and requested that her husband should be able to assist her death without fear of criminal charges being brought against him. She took her case through the legal system up to the House of Lords and on to the European Court of Human Rights. It was her need for assistance which made Diane Pretty's case one which entered the ground of assisted suicide. A request for the withdrawal of treatment would have been quite another matter.

On 29 April 2002 Diane Pretty lost her case. Ten days later she died in a hospice: her condition had deteriorated and she had developed the respiratory problems which she had feared and which had prompted her request. It is one of life's ironies that on the day that Diane Pretty received the European Court's verdict, Ms B – a paralysed woman who had requested withdrawal of her life support – died in her sleep having been granted her request (Boyd 2002: 211). This on the face of it looks like an unfairness: two bodies being treated differently, their owners being given differing control over their destiny. Morally one might argue that the cases are similar: two forty-three-year-old women wanting to end their lives, both in need of help to effect their wishes. However, the legalities and indeed the wider social context and ramifications make the cases different.

The difference in legal terms is that Diane Pretty was requesting her husband's help, whereas Ms B was asking that treatment be withdrawn. Ms B, a competent adult, was within her rights to ask for withdrawal. The British Medical Association guidance says:

> The right of competent adults to refuse treatment was re-affirmed in the 1998 case of *St George's Healthcare NHS Trust* v. *S* in which the court held competent adults have the absolute right to refuse medical treatment ... even if they might die as a result of that refusal. (2001: 17)

Diane Pretty's request was that she could be assisted to die with dignity. She did not want to await the natural trajectory of her devastating illness, nor did she wish to die as a result of the withdrawal of the tube through which she was fed.

Taking a moral approach to these cases, it is not so easy to make the distinction. Whilst the legal position remains firm on the question of taking life, it has changed over the years from a rigid no to any life-shortening measures to a position where under certain circumstances these are allowed, as we have seen in the Quinlan and Bland judgements. If we take a more sociological approach, we would perhaps have to take account of the wider effects of this act by an individual. Involving others in assisted suicide starts to move away from the accepted norms that society adheres to in terms of respect for life. The nature of relationships between family members may be at risk of change and go on to produce a less functional society as a whole. Singer says that while the distinction between the Diane Pretty and Ms B cases which was made at law 'may accurately state the law that governs these situations, it does not rest on a defensible moral basis' (2002: 234).

Ms B had been ventilated following the rupture of a blood vessel in her neck which left her paralysed from the neck down. She was deemed by the medical staff to be mentally competent and had repeatedly requested that the ventilator support be withdrawn. The British Medical Association's ethical guidelines are clear on the fact that 'a voluntary refusal of life-prolonging treatment by a competent adult must be respected' (2001: 15). However, the doctors argued that until Ms B had a chance to attempt rehabilitation, she could not make an informed decision about withdrawal. The doctors also argued that they would not switch off the ventilator because they had come to know and respect Ms B (*Bulletin of Medical Ethics* 2000: 5). If this overriding of rights is to be the result of empowered patients, improved communication and a partnership where there is respect between doctor and patient, one could be forgiven for hankering after good old-fashioned paternalism.

The President of the Family Law Division of the High Court, Dame Elizabeth Butler-Sloss, went to Ms B's bedside. In judging in her favour Butler-Sloss noted that patients that were mentally competent but physically disabled had the same rights to autonomous decision making as any other mentally competent person (2000: 6). In comparing the two cases Singer (2002) says that a lay observer would say the judgements were inconsistent, whereas a lawyer would recognise the two principles upon which they were based: the right to refuse medical treatment and the prohibition on assisting suicide. Technically the lawyers, Singer argues, are correct, but

> in a deeper ethical sense, the lay observers are right. We have arrived at the absurd situation where a paralysed woman can choose to die when she wants if her condition means that she needs some form of medical treatment to survive; whereas another paralysed woman cannot choose to die when or in the manner she wants, because there is no medical treatment keeping her alive in such a way that if it were withdrawn, she would have a humane and dignified death. (2002: 234)

Singer suggests that these different legal arguments have led to contradiction and that the answer lies in moving away from a rule-based ethics and thinking about the consequences of actions.

The withdrawal of ventilation is usually thought of in the cases of head injury and, as we have seen, one of the problems is the difficulty of knowing what the patient would have wanted. In the course of the interviews with ICU nursing staff in my study, there were discussions about the removal of ventilators in cases where, owing to chronic lung conditions, patients could only manage a few breaths on their own. These patients are fully aware and had been fully in agreement with the decision, recognising that their quality of life was just too poor for them to wish to go on.

In one interview with two senior intensive care nurses, the discussion turned to the withdrawal of treatment for patients who are fully alert and aware of their circumstances. These are patients with chronic obstructive airways disease who are ventilator dependent and despite all efforts cannot be weaned off the machine. Sometimes the most humane line of treatment is to withdraw the ventilator and see how things turn out. Here the nurses cite two very different cases. What comes through the discussion is the very matter-of-factness about the way things are in the last few days for these patients. This in no sense represents an uncaring approach, and nor is a critical comment intended on my part; it is merely a commentary on the nature of life when, in the absence of medical technology, the body is quite simply past fixing.

The first case is unexpectedly successful:

LP: Yes because there have been a few, especially chronic obstructive airways disease, who have looked black when you have been trying to wean them, very poor, and the decision is taken, we just extubate and let nature take its course, if God wants these people to breathe they will breathe, and they come to see you ten days later and they are going home. At one point you were thinking, just pull the tube, pull the screens, a bit of diamorph if they get harassed, keep them comfy, and they come with a box of chocolates when they are on their way out the door, wow!

In the second example that the nurses gave the patient did not do so well. Interestingly the focus is still on the everyday, even though they know, as does the patient, that death is near:

BL: And we have had other people, usually they are awake they are on the ventilator. We had one lady it was her birthday, she had her family ...
LP: chocolate cake ...
BL: chocolate cake, chocolates in the night, knowing that the next day, that the tube was going to get pulled, they were not going to get re-intubated. Essentially they know that when that tube comes out they are unlikely to survive, these are people who are awake and conscious.
LP: Yes, that was a difficult one.
BL: I think that happened on at least one other occasion, you speak to these people, they are essentially like you or I, fully alert in the bed, just the fact that they are on the ventilator, but they know that it is the end of the road and that tomorrow they will be

kept comfortable and that is it.

Let us return to the beating-heart donor. How is it possible to behave towards a human body in a way which does not square with Kant's exhortation to treat people as ends in themselves and not as means to an end? Answers to this question are to be found beyond the immediate demands of the donor body. There is the idea that good can come of a death, and an altruistic act to offer another person a chance of life is the motivation behind what in other circumstances would be thought of as body snatching. Porter notes that advances in technology bring with them moral worries:

> In the United States Dr H. Barry Jacobs floated the International Kidney Exchange with a view to importing Third World kidneys for sale to American citizens. Executed criminals in China already have organs harvested; kidney sales by poor people have become common in various developing countries and are not unknown in Harley Street. (1997: 625)[6]

The practice of organ donation via the elective ventilation of a brain dead person can be upheld by reference to beneficence. The argument is that once the possibility of life has ceased for the donor body, the question of non-maleficence does not seriously arise and the overwhelming case is for beneficence with regard to the organ recipient. The strength of this conviction is evidenced in the fact that some countries uphold an opt-out policy for organ donation with the presumption being that organs are available unless stated otherwise.

We can also point to quite distinct futures for the recipient and donor bodies. The recipient body, after receiving the organ from the donor, will be for some time dependent upon the skills of an anaesthetist and the skills and teamworking of an intensive care team. Unlike the donor body, which will go on to be buried or cremated, this body will, if all goes to plan, revert to a fully autonomous functioning state. The point I am making is that the day to day care of the bodies will not appear too dissimilar. All the while these bodies possess characteristics that would cause us to categorise them as bodies. Yet in functional, clinical and, arguably, moral terms they differ.

PERSON–BODY CONTINUUM

In terms of the physical care involved, we can think of a continuum with the body at one end and the person at the other. The meaning that the body carries when it is in a fully autonomous and conscious state differs from that carried by the unconscious body or by the body in persistent vegetative state, or indeed when the body is being ventilated and perfused prior to providing organs for transplant to another body. Even the routine patient becomes a little more body than person by virtue of becoming a patient. Health care professionals may like to deny this, but if it were not the case that the body as a purely physical entity is the focus some of the time, I doubt that it would be so necessary for them to remind themselves and their students that 'patients are people'. Towards the extreme body end of this body–person continuum is the 'beating-heart donor', where the patient has become much more of a body, in fact a provider of organs for transplantation. In caring for the donor prior to transplant surgery, the main task is to maintain the organs in a state of readiness for transplant. The health care professionals, and most particularly the nurses, find themselves working in very ambiguous territory.

The public outcry at the scandal concerning hospital pathology departments' retention of body parts without parental consent led to a complete rethink of the way the health service relates to bodies and the rights of relatives in this area. The Redfern Report (2001) revealed that at Alder Hey Hospital pathologists had removed at post-mortem and retained 2,080 organs from 800 children. One pathologist, since banned from practice in the UK, was largely responsible. However, a survey across the UK revealed that large collections of organs were retained in hospitals and medical schools. The inquiry prompted changes in the law, and perhaps more importantly in the culture with regard to informed consent. A commission was set up to oversee the return of body parts to parents. There was a spate of press coverage of parents holding separate burial services for the returned body parts, these sometimes taking place years after the original funeral.

These very public inquiries led to a call for more openness. There were also unexpected consequences for the supply of organs: the willingness to consent to donation of organs dropped for a short period as there was confusion in the public's mind between organ retention and organ donation. It is interesting to note that in Scotland the consultation concerning organ retention and donation treated them as separate issues so that the one did not reduce donations in the other. In England and Wales the inquiry took the two issues together.

The findings of the high profile Kennedy Report (2001) on the high incidence of deaths of children after undergoing heart surgery at Bristol added to the general sense of mistrust of the medical profession.

Although the name Shipman should not be raised in connection with these other issues, it remains the case that his trial and conviction added to the angst and the medical profession's image was damaged. Shipman is a serial killer who was also a doctor.[7] The happenings at Alder Hey and Bristol were failures of individuals and systems, but negligent practices of a quite different order.

Atkinson (1995: 6), in a discussion of how much medical discourse takes place at a remove from the patients, notes how sociologists of

health and illness have tended to comment unfavourably on the dehumanising processes whereby the person becomes a patient. However, as
the person becomes a patient he or she also becomes a case. Atkinson
says the process involves a good deal of talk – talk which focuses upon
the patient, talk which is a very human activity. His point is that it is possible in describing medical practice to overstate the dehumanising case
and forget how much subjective human performance goes into the medical discourse which produces the case to be treated.

Seymour (2000: 91) picks up on Atkinson's work concerning 'reading' the body and the 'negotiated product' which is the medical knowledge of the individual: clinical data are open to various interpretations.
On Seymour's analysis of the events leading to withdrawal of treatment
in the ICU, she makes the distinction between 'bodily death' and 'technical death', the former being what appears to be happening in the bed
and the latter being how the clinical pathology analysis 'reads' the situation. As noted in Chapter 2, the point of Seymour's analysis is that for
a natural death to occur in ICU following the withdrawal of treatment,
it is important that there is no causal link between the withdrawal and
the death; rather it is important that the 'technical' reading of the body
is that it is beyond treatment and that further efforts would be futile. The
concern is to bring technical death and bodily dying into alignment
(2000: 103) so that death occurs at the right time. Much of this was discussed in Chapter 2; however, in the context of the present chapter it
points to the distinctions we have made between the biological body and
the human body.

Intensive care is often the starting point for discussions of principles
of autonomy and respect for persons. This is because it provides a high
profile context for debate and often dramatic cases. However, the analyses of the issues raised by caring for bodies – sociological and philosophical analyses – are relevant in less dramatic settings. Technological
possibilities, advances in medical science, along with societal expectations have placed intensive care medicine in a central position when it
comes to this question of the body and its meaning. There are fine lines
to be drawn between when we are dealing with a person and when we
are dealing with a body. These questions are in some ways similar to
those posed at the beginning of life as to when life begins, at ensoulment
or when the primal streak is established and so on. When the treatment
becomes futile and life has been sustained but to no avail, are we really
talking about life or death? At some level, nursing care is about looking
after the body whatever the medical treatment or nursing management
of care. This remains true when treatment is limited, withheld or withdrawn. Nursing is the health care profession charged with caring –
doing, according to Henderson's (1960) unmatched definition, what
patients would do for themselves if they were able. Whether a nurse is
following the consequences of a medical decision to treat, or a legal deci-

sion to continue or withdraw, it is the person in that role, the nursing role, who is handling the micro-level detail of major value judgements.

FEEDING THE BODY

Feeding is a central issue in this whole question of caring for bodies. In situations where health care professionals are continuing to manage cases where there is no treatment to offer and no prospect of recovery, the main carers involved are the nurses. In cases where it has been decided to withdraw treatment, there are often residual difficulties over the matter of feeding. The question here is often an emotional one, but it is the case with ethical issues that however much we may defer to philosophical positions and try to apply ethical principles, there is an element of gut-level emotion that enters into the debate. Whilst I would not suggest that we follow the gut and abandon the moral philosophy, I would argue that it is not wise to ignore the more basic emotional instincts. Nurturing the patient, providing basic needs of food and drink, is held by many to be at the heart of nursing care. Although there is research evidence that nutritional requirements are often not met by hospital catering (McWhirter and Pennington 1994), the image of the nurturing and caring profession is strong.

As we saw in the last chapter, a question which is frequently raised is whether feeding by artificial means should be regarded as a treatment and thereby open to discontinuation when the prognosis is poor. This matter may well have been settled at law, but it leaves ethical niggles in the minds of many. This is a particularly sensitive issue for nurses as they are the members of the health care team whose responsibility it is to feed. The British Medical Association guidelines on withdrawal state:

> In England and Wales proposals to withdraw artificial nutrition and hydration from a patient who is in persistent vegetative state, or in a state of very low awareness closely resembling PVS, currently require legal review. (2001: para 21.1)

This was seen by the House of Lords as an interim measure. In discussion of this guide the BMA notes that this comes from the Bland case, and was based on the understanding that nutrition and hydration constituted medical treatment and to continue their provision would go against the patient's interests. The BMA position is that:

> as expertise and professional guidelines develop on persistent vegetative state, the BMA can see no reason to differentiate between decisions for patients in PVS and those for patients with other serious conditions where artificial nutrition and hydration are not considered to be a benefit, which are currently governed by established practice without the need for legal review. (2001: 63)

In Scotland there is no requirement to go to court in arriving at a decision to withdraw artificial nutrition and hydration. There is, then, the possibility of prosecution if the Court of Session has not granted authority.[8]

Zussman (1992: 177) makes a point about the difference between what the law says and its effects on human action. He is taking up Weber's distinction (in *Economy and society*, 1922) between a legal and a sociological concept of the law. A similar distinction can be drawn in this case where the law is clear but the sociological analysis reveals that there is a good deal of moral disquiet around the decisions taken according to the legal position. Singer's (2002) analysis of the Ms B and Diane Pretty legal decisions would be an example of this.

Sociology's fascination with the body is of interest to health care professionals; it is also arguably a source of curiosity. Whilst sociology, as we have noted, is concerned that the discipline has not taken sufficient interest in the body, it has long been very much the business of those working in the health trades. So in the eyes of health care professionals, to single out the body for special treatment seems rather an odd thing to do. In medical circles the body is regarded primarily in clinical and pathophysiological terms. Nursing takes this lead to some extent, but has focused on the matter of care and on assisting patients and clients with the business of day to day living. Lawler (1991) says that the medical model deals overtly with the body but does so in a reductionist, mechanistic and deterministic way, stressing cause and effect. By contrast she notes that nursing practice is

> more interactive, more social, and more holistic. One cannot simply nurse the body in the bed. One must do business with it as a person because nursing means being able to view the body and the person as inseparable. (1991: 34)

It is hard to argue with this position and it is widely held. However it does not take us very far beyond pious hope and assertion and, perhaps worse, it shows little understanding of the medical predicament, namely, the expectation that the medical staff will come up with diagnosis and appropriate treatment. The medical model with its cause and effect and a little determinism is probably appropriate given the expectations of medicine. Either way the stereotyping of one professional group by another does not bode well for teamworking in health care. There is clearly a division of labour in health care: diagnosis and treatment are the business of medicine whilst caring and co-ordination of activity around the patient are the nursing input. It is important that we do not so ossify this division that it only allows the view that it is the nursing profession that takes account of the person in the patient. Following the dichotomy we have found around the question of the patient as person or body, it would be unhelpful to arrive at a point where medicine were seen as the fixer of the biological body whilst nursing concerned itself with the human body.

WHEN THE BODY IS PAST FIXING

It is true that in the medical and nursing curricula and in those of other health care professionals there is coverage of psychosocial concerns and a good deal of discussion of the moral and legal aspects of care. The social as well as the medical approach to health and illness is well recognised. Much of the daily practice of health care has to do with effecting clinical possibilities in socially acceptable ways, in other words fitting the two models together. Nevertheless, it can be argued that, at heart, medicine is about fixing bodies. An important substantive issue for this chapter is a consideration of the question of what happens when the body is past fixing, when it can no longer function as an entity conscious of itself and in control of its life. This question leads out of some of the discussion in Chapter 2 concerning the withdrawal of feeding and treatment where their continuation are held to be clinically and morally futile. It also opens up more general debates on ethical issues in intensive care and health care more widely. As we saw in Chapter 2, the debates in moral philosophy and health care ethics focus upon the question, among others, of whether there is a difference between withdrawal and withholding of treatment. Approaching the question from a sociology of the body perspective has shed little light on the issues surrounding withdrawal of treatment and feeding. There was more promise in the contribution that law and moral philosophy have made to the 'brain death' debates.

Let us return to the idea of the continuum ranging from the completely autonomous person at one end, to the body which is not amenable to treatment on clinical or moral grounds at the other. These states can only be understood or indeed realised in a social context. Social construction has its place and its limits. The social meaning of the body clearly differs from situation to situation along this theoretical continuum.

It is also clearly difficult for relatives and friends as they are acquainted with the 'person' rather than the 'patient' or 'case', and so the further progression to 'body' is hard. At the end point of the continuum, where the person is a cadaver donor for transplant or medical education or research purposes, the 'body' status is well advanced. Even to experienced clinical minds, this is very different territory for health care professionals. The body as opposed to the person is possibly the distinction which makes health care professionals able to sustain their work in difficult cases where there is really nothing to be done in terms of cure and little to be said in terms of life.

If we can regard the body as a *person* when the brain continues to function and as a *biological entity* when brain death has occurred, we can see why the issue of withdrawal of treatment and feeding is central to nursing. Persons can act and think for themselves to varying degrees depending upon their state of health; the biological body cannot. It is when the body has failed and cannot act that continuation of treatment and sometimes feeding becomes an issue. Nursing defines itself, by and large, in terms of acting for people when their bodies will not function sufficiently for them to act alone. Health care professionals do not normally refer to the bodies that they 'fix' as bodies. They are patients, and under ideal conditions they are self-motivating, autonomous beings with rights to treatment, care, dignity and respect. When for one reason or another they are no longer autonomous and the *person* becomes more of a *body* – a failing body – the uncertain area between life and death is entered. Persistent vegetative state is, as we have seen, a classic example of this difficulty.

So does the sociology of the body have anything to offer here? My stance on the sociology of the body literature is perhaps rather sceptical in terms of what such analysis offers, beyond some rather circular, if neat, arguments. However, it does point very clearly to the fact that for human beings to function as independent autonomous actors, a functioning body is a prerequisite. Moreover, it highlights the dilemmas faced by those charged with caring for bodies which have lost their capacity for action and autonomous planning of their lives. It leads us perhaps to look upon the body with new eyes. In fact as we go about our daily lives it is difficult to associate the actions, thoughts and emotions that we undertake and experience with the organs of our body, let alone with the minute cellular activity and complexities of homeostasis and finely tuned endocrine activity, the physiology of our bodies. It is perhaps little wonder that medicine has a tendency to retreat at least for some of the time to the shelter of physiology rather than encompass the whole person.

The focus on the body seems such an obvious point but like any other taken-for-granted it sounds obvious until we come upon a case when it does not work and causes us to question the concept of body. In the case of failed bodies, bodies which are beyond treatment, the focus on the body forces a reconceptualisation of 'body'. The central question is then: what is a body? Is what we have a human being inside a body? If so, when the body ceases to work, what do we do with the human being? And importantly, who decides? And what of the body? Does the body ever become property which is separate from the human being? Mason and McCall Smith state that:

> because my body is my own, I 'own' my body. However, it is far from clear that there is support for this in either legal or ethical

terms. No ethical principle or imperative exists in which one can ground a property right in oneself. (1999: 485)

They go on to note that: 'The Human Organ Transplants Act 1989 says nothing about property in organs as such and merely criminalises those who would attempt to trade in the material' (1999: 485).

SCANDALS AND THE BODY

There have been items in the press which highlight the difficulty over the meaning and appropriate treatment of bodies. The Ice Man found in the Oetztal Valley is on display in the museum in Bolzano in the Italian Tyrol (*The Guardian* 1999). He was a human being, like you and me, and around 5,300 years ago he sat down and died of exposure and exhaustion. He is very much a body now in his own refrigerator on public display. What is it that causes us to think that this archaeological activity is justified? Is the passage of time sufficient ground upon which to make the decision that this body is no longer owed respect? The body is not property and so cannot be stolen. Again, the artist jailed for removing body parts from the anatomy museum of the Royal College of Surgeons in London was charged with theft.[9] This charge was possible because the ruling was that the parts which he took to incorporate in his art works had 'use and value' and could therefore be said to have been stolen.

Body snatching is not of course new, and the history of the medical discipline of anatomy not only is linked with art but has rather darker connections with grave robbing and worse. Porter describes this in a clear, if lurid, way:

> Brisk demand for bodies to dissect but lack of an adequate legal supply had ensured good business for the 'resurrectionists' who robbed new graves to sell their spoils to anatomists ... In 1827 an old man died in William Hare's (1792–1870) boarding-house. Hare hit upon the idea of direct selling to anatomists, bypassing the grave altogether. Spurred on by success, they turned next to murder, luring in and suffocating them, so that the corpse betrayed no trace of violence. Sixteen were done to death and their bodies sold, fetching around £7 each, before Burke and Hare were brought to justice in 1829. (1997: 317)

As a result of the outrage the Anatomy Act was passed in 1832. This Act, according to Porter, 'over the protests of a public distrustful of anatomists, awarded the medical profession the rights to "unclaimed bodies" – in effect, paupers without family dying in workhouses and hospitals' (1997: 318).

Burke and Hare, renowned in Edinburgh, were charged with outraging public decency. Public decency or at least sensibility is very much to the point here, as it is difficult to mount a case that actual harm has been done to the Ice Man or by the artist. However, public sensibility should not be taken lightly, for at least two reasons. First, it is upon a general sense of decency and sensitivity to others that much of the trust which we place in health care professionals rests. Basic, decent human values concerning what is acceptable in a civilised society very much form the bedrock of the society's morals and by extension those of its professions. Secondly, if public sensibility or sense of decency is outraged, this has knock-on effects for the professions as the basis of trust is destabilised and there can be far-reaching consequences. As Zussman (1992: 228) has it, medicine is on the decline in terms of both cultural and political authority.

As we have noted, events surrounding the Alder Hey Hospital gave rise to the unintended consequences of spurious links being made between organs being donated for transplant and retention of organs at post-mortem by pathologists. The effect was short lived in terms of organ donation, but a longer lasting effect on trust in medicine and the public's attitude led to a shortage of pathologists. If the public attitude to medicine becomes hostile the profession will in the long run become less popular, and in the short run defensive and conservative practice will result. This is not, in the round, in the best interests of patients. League tables for example listing performance in surgery will cause surgeons to fight shy of difficult cases; again this is not in the interests of patients. The quite proper call for openness, league tables and so on, if not handled well, works in the long run against the interests of society. The health care professions are not above the law, but professional self-regulation with sufficient external scrutiny is an important means of maintaining standards of quality and safety. We need to work towards maintaining standards and not take such a black and white approach to 'good surgeon, bad surgeon'. It makes no sense to act as if those down the league table can be removed and replaced. Rosenthal in her book *The incompetent doctor* (1995) shows how there is a range of possibilities before arriving at a verdict of incompetent. The ideal situation is for good professional regulation set alongside systems for quality improvement.

THE BODY AND HEALTH CARE PRACTICE

Individual action and the constraints within which it takes place are one of the central concerns of sociology. Shilling (1993) points out that the debate about the relationship between structure and agency has taken precedence over that about the relationship between mind and body. The structure or agency question concerns whether it is the structures and institutions in society which influence our actions or whether human agency – what we do – is paramount. This returns us to the question of what the body means.

Let us consider the ways in which bodies are regarded in health care practice. Even the fully independent patient loses a certain degree of autonomy by virtue of being in hospital. Zussman (1992) says that the patient disappears completely in the ICU and returns as numbers (parameters, blood gases). He says that the doctor–patient relationship is replaced by principles, patients' rights and the doctrine of informed consent. As Zussman puts it: 'the patient reappears not as a distinctive personality so much as the more or less abstract embodiment of rights' (1992: 81).

There is always a 'next of kin' (in the legal sense). There is also someone who acts as intermediary between the outside world and the patient, and who may or may not be next of kin. This person, usually a close relative or friend, may be given information, status reports after surgery for example, ahead of the patient themselves. Even enquiries over the telephone yield some general comment whilst the person in question is still asleep. This is in spite of the fact that health care professionals talk a lot about individual autonomy, the patient as an individual and individualised care. Given all of this concern with the individual, it is surprising how often this rhetoric is overridden when it comes to management of information about clinical progress.

As the patient moves along the body–person continuum they enter into a state where they are not able to make decisions about their health. As we have seen, consent to treatment becomes an issue, and questions arise of rights, proxy consent, the legal position and so on. Legal and moral debate here ranges widely, but the practical issue is about how clinicians must arrive at a course of action which would fit with the person's wishes were they able to express them.

Further still along the continuum there is death, and the person moves to the body end of the continuum. Zussman (1992: 139) argues that the law has taken over what in the past was the province of medicine. The President's Commission concerned with medical decisions makes it plain that:

> Respect for the self-determination of competent patients is of special importance in decisions to forgo life-sustaining treatment because different people will have markedly different needs and concerns during the final period of their lives ... A process of collaborating and sharing information and responsibility between care givers and patients generally results in mutually satisfactory decisions. Even when it does not, the patient's interests in self-determination and honoring the patient's own view of well-being warrant leaving with the patient the final authority to decide. (1982: 44)

In this context Zussman (1992) has a rather stark quotation from one of the physicians in his study: the remark came up in a discussion about who makes the decision to continue or not with treatment. Zussman argues that doctors have relinquished the right to make the moral judgements whilst they have reserved the technical decisions to themselves. In other words, doctors do not claim the moral expertise to say what should be done, but they do reserve the right to pronounce on the technical medical matters and so do in the end retain the power and control in the situation. As one resident physician in Zussman's study says, 'dead is when the doctors say she's dead' (1992: 149).

PERSPECTIVES ON THE BODY

Patients in persistent vegetative state are existing through their own cardiovascular efforts and so present a different legal and moral body compared with the body which is brain dead and being ventilated artificially. In either case the individuals described have in many ways become more of a body than a person; however the care and clinical decision making continue in terms of patients' best interests. The daily practice routines of care and observation of the health care professionals would appear to be the same as for any patient. In other words, the practice continues as if there were no change in the patient status, yet the health care professionals are aware of the changing bodily and moral status of the patient.

The differing perceptions of the body depend, as we have seen, on the extent to which the body is overtly inhabited by an autonomous person. These perceptions are reflected, not surprisingly, in the language we use to describe the body. Patient (client even) is the descriptor used for those being treated or cared for. Even when life is being artificially maintained the status of patient prevails. When death occurs the patient starts to be thought of as a body; the status of body becomes clearer in the postmortem room and even more so in the dissection room. The term used here is 'cadaver', from the Latin *cadere*, meaning 'to fall' (dead). The work being done on these bodies is technically similar. The psychosocial aspects will clearly differ, but what of the feelings and perceptions of the health care professionals?

Language is important in this area, as it is the way in which we give meaning to the situation. Goffman's (1969) analysis of social life divided into front regions and back regions, allowing for – to use a stage analogy – back stage and front stage behaviour, is useful here. It may be proper for one style of language to be used in the transplant theatre, but for another to be required for communication with the patient's relatives. The style of communication between health care professionals and relatives does not alter after the fact of the death in so far as reference to the deceased is concerned. Even when permission for donor organs is being sought, the person is referred to by name and there is no sense of a status transition having been made to body, let alone cadaver.

This is not to say that the language used behind the scenes, when the patients cannot hear, is always what one might term politically correct. The need to let off steam and defuse tense situations leads to a certain amount of black humour in the intensive care unit. One senior nurse in my study of ethics in intensive care spoke about a discussion that the ICU staff had been having following a patient's death. The general tone of the talk had upset a student who was new to the unit and so was not used to the culture which allowed this cynical humorous approach to breaking down tension. The ICU nurse was herself, she remembered, rather chastened by the comments of the student as she had thought that the staff were being rather restrained in deference to the student's presence.

Black humour is also found in the operating theatres. Chambliss (1996), in a dark passage in his fieldnotes, has an account of a particularly tense few minutes in the operating theatre during emergency abdominal surgery. The problem turned out to be an ectopic pregnancy.[10] The surgeon is trying to find the cause of the painful abdomen when the tube ruptures and releases the foetus. Chambliss's notes read:

> with the surgeons groping around trying to feel where things were, out of this popped up, right out of the patient and literally onto the sheet covering her, the 16-week foetus itself. Immediately one surgeon said mock-cheerfully, 'It's a boy.' 'God, don't do that,' said the scrub tech, turning her head away. (1996: 53)

The fieldnotes go on to recount how order was restored once the tension had passed, and how upset had been caused to one member of the team who did not find the black humour helped in the situation. Fox (1957; Fox and Swazey 1974) has written about the function of humour in the medical context: 'A telling sign of the tension physicians experience ... is their tendency toward counter-phobic gallows-humor jokes about how impotent they are in dealing with patients' illnesses and impending death' (1974: 62).

So what about situations where treatment and feeding are withdrawn? It is important here to consider the ways in which the body is characterised by health care professionals. As technological possibilities in health care expand, they bring with them ethical questions about the status of the body. Issues which confront the health care professionals become increasingly complex, especially for those whose business it is to care for bodies – alive, dying or, in many respects, dead. Nurses are the care workers who have the most prolonged and intimate contact with bodies. The way in which we conceptualise the body is central to much of the work carried out with bodies in the transition between life and death.

Seymour (2000) describes 'nursing care only' in the context of intensive care as something of a paradox. She talks of how nurses 'fashion their work with dying people in intensive care, investing meaning and purpose into a potentially contradictory aspect of their role' (2000: 106). This is a view of nursing in ICU consistent with that of Zussman (1992), who says that nurses have little opportunity to follow their interest in the emotional human side of care in the technologised, medically driven setting of the ICU.

In situations where treatment is withdrawn it is often the case that it makes sense to discontinue feeding, because to continue would defeat the aim of the cessation of treatment, in order to allow a more peaceful and dignified death. As we have noted, feeding is such a basic human caring activity it raises emotional as well as ethical responses.

Conceptualisation of the body is something that practitioners in health care do but they would not think of it in such terms, or at least not in the daily round of clinical life. Giddens's idea of sequestration of sickness and death may be a useful trick for society as a means of, as he puts it, 'removing basic aspects of life experience, including especially moral crises, from the regularities of day-to-day life established by the abstract system of modernity' (1991: 156). But it has to be remembered that there is a price to pay for this, and those involved in the sequestrated areas pay it. In this case the area is health care, and those working in it must find ways of incorporating the difficult aspects of this work into their day to day lives. This is true both for their work life and that outside of it. Being able to sustain a balanced life whilst undertaking what is at times frankly very emotionally demanding work requires not only a particular approach to work at an individual level, but also a work organisation which is supportive.

The ICU nurses I interviewed had strong ideas about collegial support (Melia 2001). Also, even when they had differences of opinion with the medical staff, they pointed to the fact that a strong team was one which could handle disagreement and survive to continue to work together. This data extract from an interview with a senior nurse working in an adult general ICU illustrates the point:

> RB: There have been times when we have say ward rounds and we discussed the withdrawal of therapy and we say let's leave it for another X period of time and the nurse at the bedside has come back and said 'oh no I really thought we would have moved and made a decision now', and I have to say to people, ultimately we as nursing staff, certainly not blithely, say 'I think we should think about withdrawing therapy' but as I say at the end of the day the consultants are the ones who say. I think it is easier to start therapy than it is to stop therapy.

He went on to say:

RB: And eh, that is something I have to highlight to myself and to colleagues, the fact that at the end of the day although we say yes I think it would be a good decision to withdraw, ultimately we are not the ones who 'the buck stops here' for.

KM: It is sometimes worth wondering what you would feel like if
...

BL: if you were placed in that actual position, and even sometimes when, you know, it is obvious what is going to happen if we don't withdraw therapy, something is going to happen, the patient is going to die anyway, but it is still a case of you know because sometimes these people go home, you know could I go home and sleep at night, thinking today I withdrew therapy, even if you knew within yourself it was the right thing to do, would I sleep soundly tonight knowing that?

We have already discussed the case of Anthony Bland. It was this case which led to a wide debate specifically about the withdrawal of nutrition and fluids. The debate went as far as the House of Lords (1994) where a Select Committee was set up to consider the use of life-sustaining treatments and euthanasia. In the case of Anthony Bland, the young man who sustained injury in a football stadium disaster, nurses were faced with a particularly long haul of care for a patient whose life was recognised by almost everyone involved, including his parents, in what was a very public case, to carry no meaning or quality. The law protects life to the extent that doctors in this case, with the consent and support of relatives and the large majority of the nursing staff, had to go to an English court to obtain permission for the withdrawal of nutrition. The Select Committee discussed many issues but failed to come up with a unanimous view on the central question about the withdrawal of nutrition. Having stated that 'we do not therefore distinguish between withholding and withdrawal of treatment, in our discussion of treatment limiting decisions', the Lords went on to say that:

> Treatment limiting decisions in respect of an incompetent patient should be taken jointly by all those involved in his or her care, including the entire health care team and the family or other people closest to the patient. Their guiding principle should be that a treatment may be judged inappropriate if it will add nothing to the patient's well-being as a person.

However, when it came to the issue of defining artificial means of feeding, the committee sidestepped the question, saying:

> Nor do we think it helpful to attempt a firm distinction between treatment and personal care, implying that the former may be limited and the latter not. The two are part of a continuum, and such boundary as there is between them shifts as practice evolves and particularly as the wider role of nursing develops. This boundary

is one which the courts were required to try to define in the case of Tony Bland, and that gave rise to much debate about whether nutrition and hydration, even when given by invasive methods, may ever be regarded as a treatment which in certain circumstances it may be inappropriate to initiate or continue.

In one of the less useful passages in the whole report, they say that:

> This question has caused us great difficulty, with some members of the Committee taking one view and some another, and we have not been able to reach a conclusion ... We consider that progressive development and ultimate acceptance of the notion that some treatment is inappropriate should make it unnecessary to consider the withdrawal of nutrition and hydration, except in circumstances where its administration is in itself evidently burdensome to the patient.

It is interesting to note that in the area in which the Lords had most difficulty, that is over the question of definition of artificial feeding, they introduce the developing role of the nurse as part of their argument for not distinguishing between treatment and care. It is not altogether clear what significance they placed on this, only that the 'wider role of the nurse' is mentioned. The focus in any case should be on the treatment or cure. It is too simplistic to regard medical treatment in one way and nursing care in another: feeding is bound to fall between the two here. The British Medical Association (2001) guidelines say that food or water given by ordinary means should always be offered, but not forced if patients resist or overtly refuse. Neither, the guidelines continue, should food be 'forced upon patients for whom the process of feeding produces an unacceptable level of burden, such as where it causes unavoidable choking or inspiration of food or fluid' (2001: 10). In the case of artificial nutrition and hydration being withdrawn, the BMA guidelines suggest care must be taken to document the rationale for decisions about fluids and nutrition. Cases should be reviewed by senior clinicians and the whole business be within the framework of audit and clinical governance.

There are a number of dichotomies running through this chapter. The most obvious one is the duality of mind and body which pervades the work in the area of sociology and the body. Perhaps more fundamental still is the structure and agency issue. I do not share Shilling's difficulty with Giddens's formulation, and it may be a rather simplistic notion, but I have long thought that as structure is not going to go away and social construction and individual agency can only take us so far, the reconciliation of the two within the theory of structuration (Giddens 1977) is to be welcomed.

The similarities in the philosopher's and the sociologist's approaches to the study of ethics suggest that it may be useful to utilise both perspectives, rather than to take the view that one must adopt either the philosophical argumentation method or a thoroughgoing ethnography and sociological analysis (Jennings 1990). There is a place for a clear philosophical analysis of the issues involved in withdrawal of treatment. These issues, which start out as clinical issues, have to be understood in the wider context of society. The body as person, the body as a source of organs for transplantation, the body as property, are questions which lead to wider debates concerning moral, legal, economic and ultimately political questions. As we have seen, the need to produce a legal definition of death led to some distinctions being made with respect to the body, the most useful one to my mind being to think in terms of human life and bodily life.

The focus of this chapter has been the caring for bodies, whatever their status and whatever questions they raise for health care professionals. My aim in this book is to further the case for a health care ethics that focuses on the patient rather than approach the matter in terms of medical ethics, nursing ethics and so on. That said, it is often argued that the moral dilemmas and issues which arise in patient care present different problems for the different professional groups, and this is then the rationale for separate approaches to ethics. One important point that can be made from the perspective of the nursing profession is that nursing is often in the position of being obliged to follow the decisions and to cope with the consequences, foreseen and unforeseen, of those decisions. In medical decisions to treat, to withdraw, to treat this way or that, nurses are consulted but the decision is ultimately a medical one. Likewise, decisions taken in the law courts that treatment may or may not be discontinued have consequences for nurses, as they will be the most closely involved with the patient care.

This line of argument is beginning to sound like a rationale for the separate nursing and medical approaches to ethics for health care, but this is not my intention. My comments do not constitute a complaint on behalf of nurses: they are merely a statement of fact in a situation where the medical profession, after due consultation with other professionals and patients, and where appropriate their relatives, takes the decisions. When the doctors feel that they may not be on secure moral and legal grounds, the law is called upon. It is a symptom of advanced medical practice that situations will arise where we have to ask the legal profession for assistance in arriving at just care. If we are to make the case for health care ethics, with the patient at centre stage, it is important that the different professions involved understand one another and can see the issue from each other's perspective in order to arrive at agreement on the best way to proceed. For this to happen we need to be able to analyse the situation from various angles and separate out the arguments before building back up to a whole. This question of approach to health care ethics for the health caring professions is taken up in the next chapter.

NOTES

1   The terms 'medical sociology' and 'sociology of health and illness' are used interchangeably throughout the book.

2   The BSA annual conference in 1998 took as its theme 'making sense of the body'. A selection of papers from that conference can be found in Backett-Milburn and McKie (2001).

3   Peter Singer (1994: 57) provides a very clear and sensitive account of these cases.

4   See also Mason and McCall Smith (1999: 396–7, 409–10).

5   *Airedale NHS Trust* v. *Bland* 19 February 1993, 2, *Weekly Law Reports*, p. 350.

6   Harley Street is the UK's renowned concentration of private medical practice.

7   www.the-shipman-inquiry.org.uk.

8   *Law Hospital NHS Trust* v. *Lord Advocate* 1986.

9   Society.Guardian.co.uk, 31 October 2002.

10   A particularly dangerous situation where the foetus is developing in the Fallopian tube; this presents with acute pain and the mother is in danger of haemorrhage.

V from teamwork to ethics

WG: Probably he should have died the weekend I had him but a doctor chose to resuscitate him ...

MV: His blood pressure was no good and terrible and the consultant on the ward round said no we have to do everything. I said right OK, I am going to be on your back every second of this morning and every second of the day, because I am fed up of every doctor saying that to me. I said you do half-heartedness and then you just walk away and leave him and nobody does anything, so I will be on your back every five seconds about what is happening to this man ...

It was like an exodus from the bed space, they [the surgeons on the ICU] never came near the bed, didn't want to know what was happening, didn't really want to at all. Didn't want to get involved so they didn't. (senior nurses cardiac ICU)

TJ: I can remember one poor lady with profound ARDS [acute respiratory distress syndrome] and on the Sunday night eventually saying to the consultant, 'Look – I had been on holiday for two weeks – nothing has changed, in fact things are worse than before I went on holiday here. The family are continuing to look for "tomorrow things are going to improve". And he got the family in at 6 p.m. on the Sunday night and sat down, and the husband knew it was coming, because this had been going on for seven weeks. And he took the decision there and then to withdraw, so that he did not have to hand it over to another consultant on Monday morning, which would have meant another three or four days to get to know the patient and it could have just dragged on and on. And I really admired him for that because he saw what I was saying and sat down and looked back in the notes and eventually said, 'look you know ... let's just see what the family think' ...

So I think you know, when things have become ethically difficult, morally difficult, they [the doctors] will listen to what we have to say. As we said already, legally the buck stops with them, we can put our arguments but at the end of the day we just have to accept what comes. (senior nurse ICU)

These extracts from the interview data in my study of ethics in intensive care illustrate the main arguments of the book. They show the importance of context. Also, the extracts demonstrate that whilst there is disagreement and difficulty between doctors and nurses in the ICU there is also a strong sense of team and that this persists even when the going gets rough. When it is only the nursing input that is required to meet the patient need in the end stages of withdrawing treatment, this too causes tensions. For nurses this is no longer 'real' intensive care and the situation can be seen in terms of bed blocking and even a squandering of intensive care expertise. However, the extracts also reveal the capacity of the team to sustain and survive quite deep divisions of opinion, even hostility. They also show how negotiation works in a situation where the medical staff can call the final shot as they are legally responsible for the decisions about treatment and clinical management.

SOCIAL ORGANISATION OF HEALTH CARE

Leaving aside the more complex analysis and cutting to the nub of the argument, here we have the idea that teamwork is the way forward for good clinical care and its attendant ethical debate. The sociological analysis of how the health care professionals operate as a group leads us to see that the straight medical dominance argument does not explain the nature of day to day practice. An examination of work practices reveals accommodation of views between the professional groups and a recognition that whilst medicine carries the legal can for decisions taken, the views of other team members, predominantly nurses, are taken into account. The sociological perspective on the organisation of care leads to a recognition that it is the nurses who provide what we might call the 'clinical civil service' of the hospital. They ensure the smooth running of the clinical units and allow the practice of medicine to take place whilst the day to day needs of patients are met and their safety and comfort ensured. This activity, generally described as care, is the province of the nursing staff.

The point of teamwork is to bring about a harmony of the care and medical activity. I am arguing that the ethical aspects of this patient management are also best approached through the kind of teamwork that we see in the ICU and so I offer it as a model for health care ethics throughout the health care system.

In this chapter I draw upon the themes and arguments made in earlier chapters in order to focus down on the case for health care ethics. As I said at the outset, health care ethics is essentially an interprofessional activity with an emphasis on the patient rather than an inward looking professional focus on medical or nursing ethics. The main idea here is that when we take a sociological approach to understanding the social practices that make up the organisation of work in the ICU, we find teamwork which depends upon a delicate balance of formal and informal rule following and breaking by which nurses manage the comings and goings of the unit and the doctors carry out medical work. With this as a starting point, the activity at the boundaries of nursing and medicine is negotiated and ways through any difficulties are found. It is my contention that this teamwork approach to the division of labour involved in patient care is equally useful when it comes to the team having to work through the moral dimension of the clinical judgements that they make in the management of patient care.

The teamwork which we find in the ICU can serve as a blueprint for the organisation and practice of care more generally. Teamwork in intensive care works because of the nature of the specialism and the condition of the patients; indeed it is difficult to envisage any other organisational system working any better. One of the main thrusts of the modernising agenda in health care in the United Kingdom is a move towards interprofessional working with a focus on the needs of the patient (Department of Health 2000). The teamwork which functions so well in the ICU suits this pattern of working. When there is a complex of diverse contributions to the total picture of patient care there needs to be a co-ordinated approach and, over time, teamwork has emerged as the dominant model for care.

HEALTH CARE ETHICS: LESSONS FROM INTENSIVE CARE

One of the lessons from the ICU which can be transported more generally into other areas of health care is that multidisciplinary teamwork has the additional benefit of being a good starting point for handling the moral dimension of care. For open discussion of the moral aspects of care, team members need to be confident in themselves and each other. Whilst the intensive care unit offers a blueprint for multidisciplinary teamwork, it also demonstrates that the intensity of the work and the co-ordination of the medical and nursing work required for a team approach mean that the team members get to know one another well. Teamwork, as evidenced in the ICU, is not just a means of organising the activities; the general team approach also spills over into a team approach to a shared ethical position, or at least an effort to arrive at one. Even where the old battlegrounds of professional boundary disputes and arguments about care versus cure persist, it is possible for teams to emerge and survive. This leads us to ask what it is about the ICU that makes teamwork a more natural occurrence than perhaps in other areas of care. In other words, are there lessons from intensive care which can be useful more generally to health care delivery and, by extension, health care ethics?

We have already noted that the existence of intensive care has an effect on the rest of the health care system. Its existence draws heavily upon resources even though some of its activities cannot be said to be cost effective. However, intensive care also exerts a more pervasive effect, it offers a dimension to care – especially at the end of life – which subtly alters our view of what is possible, what as a society we can expect of medical science, technology and health care. Intensive care has become a central focus of health care, with almost iconic status. Whilst in reality it deals with only a small percentage of the health care needs of society, it represents advance in health care, high tech possibilities, and in some unstated way it offers immortality. Numerous television hospital dramas focus on the ICU or accident departments, such that the viewing public could be forgiven for thinking that most health care settings are populated by highly vocal nursing and medical staff rushing around in theatre garb, working at high octane in an endless drama. This is clearly not the case; however, as I have said, there is mileage in taking the ICU as a model for teamwork and the team approach to ethical issues in health care. One of the reasons for doing this is that in the ICU there is a blurring of roles and an obvious common purpose brought about by the very intensity of the work.

There is a case for recognising health caring professionals as a group with a similar outlook who have a need for common ground rules for ethics. The general idea here is that no matter what the disciplinary contribution is, wherever people come from, be it medicine, nursing and so on, the ethical basis for the work is the same. The need is for ethical ground rules for the practice of health care where the focus is on the patient and the rights of patients. In other words, *a rationale for ethics in the caring professions* is the stance for all disciplines. The idea of health care ethics fits well with that of teamwork as it lays emphasis on the joint activity and the patient-focused work of the team.

I am not going as far as some would in saying that what we need is a generic health worker, because I think that there is a need for strong separate disciplines from which to move to multidisciplinary health care with interprofessional teamworking. However, there are ground rules that a variety of health care professionals could subscribe to and associate themselves with as an entity broadly defined as health care ethics. The point is that all health care professionals are at one level doing the same kind of work, which Stacey (1988) termed *people work*,[1] and so all need to pay the same kind of attention to patients' needs. And in that sense, wherever the health care professions are coming from, health care ethics can be seen as a general notion which sits well with multidisciplinary working in health care. It may well be that we are moving towards one regulatory body in professional health care (Department of Health 1999; JM Consulting 1996; 1998; Merrison Report 1975), but meantime a unity of approach to health care ethics would make a good start. Such an approach would provide a natural lead towards crossing boundaries of working practices and generally co-operating between disciplines to produce smooth running quality patient care. With health care ethics we move the focus from the professionals to patient need.

If one of the lessons from intensive care for the rest of the health service is that good practice stems from good teamwork, we still need to be clear about what we mean by teamwork and to be sure that it would travel, as it were. 'Teamwork' is a word easier said than acted out, and much ink has been spent examining the notion of teamworking. I will not rehearse the arguments here; suffice it to say that the workings of a team appear to offer the best means of providing care in a complex health service.

Teamwork in health care is recognised as a means of providing care which requires various inputs: these contributions are of different intensity and require different levels of technical and social skills. Whatever constitutes the set of skills and – to use an increasingly popular term – competencies required, it is likely to be the case that different professional and paraprofessional groups will be involved and their contributions will require to be organised and co-ordinated. This is both the strength and the problem of teamwork, for whilst it is the case that each group of health care workers has its part to play, in order to do so they have to be co-ordinated. The ground rules for the practices of working together and understanding one another's point of view can be found in intensive care. Even when there is debate and difference of opinion the aim of those involved is to arrive at best patient outcome without resorting to hierarchy or power play (Melia 2001). The working practices of those committed to teamwork provide a good basis for the same kind of joint approach to understanding and discussion that is necessary for ethical debate.

THE ORGANISATIONAL CONTEXT OF CARE

Throughout the work I have deliberately focused on a small body of literature dealing with the sociological analysis of work in hospitals and in particular in intensive care. Chambliss (1996) studied the work of nurses in order to open up a more empirically based approach to bioethics. He notes that typically bioethicists debate hypothetical cases and the result, he says, is 'intellectually challenging but not very useful' (1996: 6). By focusing on nursing Chambliss says he sought to 'move ethics from a formal individualism to a broader organisational awareness' (1996: 7).

This shift of focus comes about because Chambliss holds that:

Nursing's problems in particular reflect the organisational structures in which nurses work, and any serious discussion of ethics
in nursing must deal with these realities. In looking at nurses' ethical difficulties we necessarily learn about life in organisations.
(1996: 7)

Chambliss makes some very useful points about the nature of organisations and the joint moral enterprise of those working within them. He
says:

In nursing the old model of ethical dilemmas is becoming obso-
lete; the diffusion of responsibility makes true dilemmas less and
less common. Instead, ethical dilemmas are the moral outcrop-
pings of differences between relatively powerful groups. Ethical
problems are no longer the heavy burden of the lone practitioner,
such as the traditional physician. There are too many other parties
involved: nurses, administrators; families; lawyers ... as a multi-
plicity of constituencies inside the hospital, then, increasingly,
ethical issues entail conflicts between constituencies. In a sense,
everyone in the hospital becomes a subordinate to someone else,
then moral problems are externalised and become practical,
debatable issues of politics. Even for physicians, ethical problems
are now manifestations of conflicts with patients, families, or reg-
ulators of some sort. (1996: 94)

Here Chambliss makes the point that essentially the means of organisation of care – the hospital – becomes something of a player in how ethical issues are worked through. Organisations and their routines present
opportunities for those working in them to avoid some of the immediate
difficulties that arise in the core work of the organisation – in this case
the emotional and ethical aspects of patient care which make the work
stressful. Nurses can take refuge in routines and paperwork to gain
some respite from the stresses of being so closely involved with people's
raw emotions (Menzies 1970; Strauss 1978).

Chambliss puts it well when, in talking of the size of the hospital
organisation and the division of labour, he says they allow for denying
responsibility but also, paradoxically, for taking responsibility and using
discretion:

Vast discretion [can be] exercised, awesome choices can be made,
and yet all of it remains invisible. But even when such choices are
made, as in the choice to let a patient die, the usual effect of the
staff's handling of the death is to reinforce in their minds the place
of the organisation itself as the effective moral actor. (1996: 179)

This is an interesting view. However his analysis of the nursing profession's position of subordination, with nurses often being left out of the

decision making in clinical care, is perhaps rather dated. This leads to a rather stale rerun of the medical dominance thesis.

As we noted in Chapter 1, Chambliss's work is closely linked to the earlier work of Zussman (1992), whose study of medical ethics, as we have seen, was based in the intensive care units of two American hospitals. Zussman's work reveals much about the working practices of intensive care but also gives us insights into the medical profession and its practice. Zussman examines, among other things, the ways in which the medical profession retains control of decision making in the ICU. Whilst nursing may at times feel sidelined by medicine, the medical profession, some argue, works in the shadow of the law courts. In a world where there is a predominance of decisions driven by patients' rights and a recourse to the law for judgements upon clinical decisions, it is interesting to note the ways in which the medical profession does succeed in retaining power in this area.

What both authors show is that intensive care practice is very much culturally and socially circumscribed. Zussman and Chambliss note that the social processes and organisational factors are important if we are to understand intensive care practice. Zussman (1992) in particular shows how medicine finds ways to retain essential control of the management of patient care, especially in relation to prolonging or withdrawing treatment by being clear about what constitutes a technical medical decision. So whilst lawyers and philosophers will have views on the rights to treatment and the morality of certain courses of action, the disciplines of law and moral philosophy are not the ones to say what will or will not produce a clinical improvement. As Zussman puts it:

> when physicians do resist the wishes of patients and their families, they justify that resistance by moving decisions from the realm of values to the realm of technique. Thus, physicians argue, frequently and insistently, that some decisions are not value laden at all but simply technical. As such, many physicians argue, they are beyond the proper range not only of patients and families but of the law and ethics more generally. (1992: 141–2)

In this way Zussman says we have ethics 'transformed into medicine' (1992: 151).

Seymour (2000) too sees the importance of the organisation in treatment decisions and ethical considerations. The central theme in her study of death and dying in the ICU is that whilst ethical and scientific principles are used, they are subject to interpretation and reinterpretation. In other words the social context of a particular event is important if we are to understand what is going on in the ICU. As Seymour puts it, it is important to view the 'decision making as a social process bounded by particular organisational contexts, rather than the product of individual reasoning governed by immutable ethical and scientific principles'(2000: 155).

Professions in health care have, not unreasonably, been likened to tribes (Bucher and Strauss 1961). The strength of the loyalty to the tribe, as opposed to the team, should not be underestimated.[2] Various accounts of the organisation and workings of health care describe hospitals as locales in which professionals do their work (Etzioni 1961; 1975; Freidson 1970; 1994; Mauksch 1966; Strauss et al. 1963). Whilst there is a long tradition of adopting a power analysis approach to the relationship between medicine and nursing (Freidson 1970; Mackay 1993; Wicks 1998; Witz 1992), the idea of negotiation is more fruitful. As we have seen in intensive care the final decision may rest with the medical profession, but that fact does not wish away the importance of working relationships and the need for co-operation among ICU team members.

PROFESSIONAL INTERDEPENDENCE

Freidson in his classic *Profession of medicine* (1970) points out that doctors and other health carers for that matter cannot function alone: they depend on the division of labour and the co-operation of others. Given the long-standing tradition of a dominant medical profession taking a lead in health care, such an insight is far-reaching. As health care has become more complex the notion of medicine as a single entity is probably no longer such a useful concept. Just as we have seen the specialisms in medicine play a part in arriving at clinical decisions (Atkinson 1995), so too do the various professional and organisational inputs to the health service. The day to day smooth running of hospital wards and units, it can be said, is largely due to the work of nurses. There has to be co-operation between professional groups if the good management of patient care is to be achieved. Medical and nursing work are interdependent entities and a good deal of patient management depends upon nurses carrying out the instructions and prescriptions of medicine. It also involves medicine relying on nursing's observation and charting of patient progress. Although there is a lot of scope for boundary crossing in terms of the perimeters of each health care professional's area of practice, there are core skills and knowledge bases within each professional group. For the two main players in health care this means that medicine diagnoses and treats, whilst nursing provides the care and has experience and knowledge of the management of patients' needs during their experience of illness and dependency.

In this division of labour, nursing is dependent upon medicine for diagnosis and prescription, and in its turn medicine is dependent upon nursing for providing the care and patient support – the context in which cure is brought about, or at least the circumstances in which medicine's contribution can be made. 'Doctor's orders' is a long established phrase, patients use it. It is a phrase that suggests that the medical imperative is a force within society, even in these days when the language of rights is common in health care and when there is a good deal of health related knowledge in society (there is also a good deal of ignorance). So whilst medicine no longer occupies quite such a dominant position in society as was once the case, medical prescription still holds sway. A good deal of trust is placed in doctors, and their judgement and their clinical lead are therefore accepted. With the changes in health care practice and new working relationships being forged between the professions in health care, there is a gradual nudging aside of this medically dominated version of health care. It is likely that it will be through teamwork that the changes are made. Organisational reforms, pathways for care and 'redesigned' ways of delivering health care all depend upon teamwork (Department of Health 1998).

The occasions when the interdependence of the two professions, nursing and medicine, is a matter for debate are more often than not resolved through some compromise or team discussion. Recognition of the difficulties inherent in the relationship between nursing and medicine is not new. Florence Nightingale, in a letter to Sydney Herbert in 1855, wrote: 'It is obvious that what I have done could not have been done had I not worked with the medical authorities and not in rivalry with them' (Vicinus and Nergaard 1989). And, in her famous work *Notes on nursing* (1859) she said: 'No man, not even a doctor, ever gives any other definition of what a nurse should be than this – "devoted and obedient". This definition would do just as well for a porter. It might even do for a horse.' We have moved on, but history leaves its mark.

If we focus upon the interdependence of nursing and medicine it can be seen that a strong relationship exists when there is little in dispute either about practices and treatments or about the division of labour. In other words, when routine practices suffice, all runs smoothly. The difficulty comes where the ground is not so clear and undisputed and where the division of labour is problematic. Whichever way we look at it, the fact of the matter is that medicine carries the can for the overall plan of action for each patient. Whilst nursing might have, to its own satisfaction, made the case for a version of nursing which is independent of medicine, it is not so clear that patients have adopted that viewpoint. As teamwork becomes the norm, and hospital and primary care organisations become increasingly aware of their legal responsibilities for the provision of care, there will be more boundary blurring and some extended role taking by nurses and other health care professionals. In the patient's mind and in unspoken custom and practice understanding, it is the medical professional – general practitioner or consultant – who carries responsibility for the management of a patient's care. However, new flexible practices are accommodated by virtue of the health care organisations, hospitals and health centres having systems in place through which the patient has direct access and a right to redress if there are any problems with the nature or provision of their care. Again we see an example of the organisation as opposed to the individual clinician having clear responsibility for care. This is not to say that each professional is not also accountable at law for their own actions. It is merely symptomatic of an increasingly managed health service. This makes for interesting speculation from the standpoint of the sociology of the professions. Professions in bureaucracies have long been a topic of interest. As a health service seeks to modernise and put the patient in the centre of its enterprise, questions are raised about professional autonomy and interprofessional working practices.

The ICU is a prime area for the crossing of professional boundaries, with nursing undertaking an exceptional amount of technical work and medical staff being around the patient during much of the basic caregiving. This state of affairs is due to the concentration of clinical activity and observation that goes on around the patient. Also, the severity of the conditions of the patients in ICU means that they are constantly attended by at least one nurse and the medical staff see them on a more frequent basis than is the case in other areas of the hospital. The sheer pragmatic practicalities of two professions working so closely means that a daily blurring and crossing of roles takes place. Nurses may in general be the ones to attend to the patient's comfort and to physically move them as required, but it is not uncommon for medical staff to assist if they are on the spot when the need arises. This close proximity gives both professions a good understanding of each other's work. This is not to say that it is always a picture of sweetness and light, but despite the ups and downs of ICU life, the professional groups do get to know each other, warts and all. By experiencing their practices in such a close working situation, nurses and doctors see each other in the raw as it were, and this has the additional advantage of making a good basis for ethical debate. Colleagues may not always agree with each other but they can accept one another's point of view and understand and recognise their interdependence. My point is that if you can do teamwork you can, by following the same model, do ethics.

The social practices involved in the day to day organisation of health care, when examined through the methods of sociology, demonstrate how the team brings about care and cure. The experience of teamwork allows health care workers to air different opinions, positions and moral possibilities and to work together in a kind of ethical teamwork. The practice of teamwork exercises the communication and understanding 'muscles' needed for ethical discussion and the resolution of the ethical questions which have come to be associated with health care.

Nurses, as I have suggested, can be thought of as the 'clinical civil service' of the hospital. They enforce many of the rules of the organisation and the more senior nurses constitute a long-standing knowledgeable core staff group on units where many others – students, nurses undertaking postgraduate courses and junior medical staff – rotate. Thus just as the permanent civil servants of government provide continuity to government departments as ministers come and go, so it is in hospitals that the nursing staff provide the stability and knowledge base for the day to day delivery of health care. The role of the nurses in the maintenance of the smooth running of the hospital, the 'clinical civil service' role, can lead to problems with other professional groups involved in health care. Chambliss says that what look like ethical debates are sometimes matters of 'power and who will make the decision' (1996: 8). As we have seen in situations of withdrawal of treatment, efforts are made to come to a team decision, including the family; however it is ultimately a medical call. The nurses are then sometimes left to effect a decision which they would not have made. Chambliss says, 'what officially appears as an ethics argument is actually a thinly disguised turf battle' (1996: 8). Whether it is a 'turf' battle or genuine disagreement over a moral judgement, it is the case that intensive care requires the integrity of the team and so it has to be able to resolve disputes to move on unscathed to work together another day (Melia 2001).

It is sometimes the case that nurses will break the rules in order to maintain the smooth running of patient care. Allen describes boundary blurring, especially in the area of prescribing or the ordering of blood tests:

> There is a sense in which some blurring of the nurse–medical boundary is unavoidable. This reflects the impossibility of sustaining a formal division of labour in which doctors diagnose and nurses merely observe ... out of the wealth of information nurses gather about patients they have to decide what is medically relevant. (1997: 511)

In making this point, Allen is drawing on Gamarnikow (1991), who has noted that the medical viewpoint is necessarily mediated by nursing practice as medicine is reliant upon nursing observation.

SOCIOLOGICAL INSIGHTS AND ETHICS

Routine is one of the mainstays of hospital life and of nursing practice in particular. This is used to maintain safe practice and it allows for strangers to be cared for by strangers. Beyond routine, of course, nursing does offer all the psychosocial aspects of care. The fact that both patients and health care professionals are human beings is mapped onto the routines; care is individualised and personalised. Nonetheless, it has to be said that, as far as physical care is concerned, the business could be achieved without these emotional elements of the work. It is routine, reliable and regular safe practices that are essential for the delivery of health care.

The sociological literature on hospitals as organisations and the work presented in the earlier chapters demonstrate that it is important to locate ethical debates about health care in their clinical and social context in order to take account of the working practices and professional cultures of those involved. One of the functions of a sociological analysis of these difficult clinical situations is that it helps us to get beyond the stereotypes and the rather trite division between care and cure that is sometimes proffered, usually in order to elevate the care role of nursing. If we move beyond this we can begin to lay the ground for ethics for health care professionals.

Callahan, in a discussion entitled 'The social sciences and the task of bioethics', recalls with some delight that he learnt something from two anthropologists (Muller and Koenig 1988), something that he says he might

> never have discovered on my own, and surely not from moral philosophy: that medical residents are prone to define death not as the failure of critical bodily organs but as occurring when technological interventions no longer work – death as technological failure. (1999: 285)

This analysis is very similar to the kinds of descriptions to be found in Zussman's work. In his paper Callahan is questioning both the direction that bioethics has taken in its liking for the four principles, or 'principlism' as some would have it, and also the benefits that social science, particularly sociology, brings to bioethics. As the latter is one of the themes of this book, I draw here on Callahan's thinking on this matter.

Callahan says that he is

> uneasy with the contention that the social sciences, and particularly ethnography, offer a better way forward. This may be so but only if they are combined with a way of pursuing ethical analysis that knows how to make good use of social-science knowledge, whether quantitative or qualitative. Ethics must, in the end, be ethics, not social science. (1999: 285)

Callahan argues that there is a myth abroad that the social science analysis can provide an idea of how things are and so give a steer to how they ought to be. He calls this

> the 'is–ought fallacy': the belief that a moral 'ought' can be deduced from a factual 'is'. Not so, as most philosophers have held at least since the time of David Hume, who first called attention to it. (1999: 286)

This steer from 'is' to 'ought' is not what I would see to be the point of the sociological analysis, which brings an understanding of the social context in which moral decisions are taken in health care. As Callahan says, ethics has to be ethics, not social science. What the sociological analysis brings is an understanding of how the moral 'oughts' are sometimes difficult to arrive at because of the context of the factual 'is'. Also, the 'is' is not always so straightforwardly factual because we are dealing with various people's perspectives of a situation, multiple realities and so on. So there is always doubt, uncertainty and more than one interpretation or view. In this respect the sociological analysis is not dissimilar from the ethical analysis. Callahan (1999: 292) notes that Renée Fox's great contribution to understanding medicine is the idea of 'medical uncertainty' (we have already discussed this in Chapter 2). Sociological analysis of the workings of intensive care units reveals how some of the problems stem from the differing perspectives of a situation as well as the possible differences of moral viewpoint. Callahan notes that:

> No-one is prepared to reject medicine because it cannot get rid of that uncertainty. Bioethics is no less filled with uncertainty, and, as in medicine, the real test is the way uncertainty is handled. An unwillingness to confront it leads to evasion and rigidity in bioethics no less than in medicine. (1999: 292)

This idea of the place of applied disciplines in relation to medicine is interesting and various writers on bioethics have touched upon the theme. Hoffmaster notes that: 'Bioethics has been preoccupied with making judgements about troublesome moral problems and justifying those judgements' (2001: 1). He says that the intention of the book he edited entitled *Bioethics in social context* is to 'Show that bioethics is as much about *understanding* as it is about *justification*, and to give social scientists a prominent position in a reoriented bioethics' (2001: 1). And he goes on to say that:

> Indeed, it would seem that understanding has to accompany, if not precede, any genuine form of justification, so that, contrary to the prevailing view, what social scientists can tell us is neither independent of nor ancillary to the enterprise of bioethics. In fact, the interpretations of moral life and moral phenomena provided by social scientists reveal that a rigorous separation of the descriptive and the normative is practically untenable. (2001: 1)

Some of the writings in the area of the distinctions between social science and moral philosophical approaches to medical ethics or bioethics leave the impression that it is essentially the turf of the moral philosophers which is being trodden by social scientists. This is largely to do with the label of ethics, which carries several meanings, one being the study of morals, and in that sense it is synonymous with moral philosophy. Zussman makes a clear distinction when he talks of 'philosophical approaches to medical ethics', as distinct from 'social science approaches to medical ethics' (2000: 7). Zussman's distinction does not carry a different meaning from that conveyed by others writing in a similar vein (Callahan 1999; Jennings 1990), but put in the way that he expresses it there is more of an even-handedness about the two approaches to the study of morals issues in the practice of health care – the philosophical and the social scientific.

Zussman, in a paper entitled 'The contribution of sociology to medical ethics' (2000), characterises the approaches of sociology and moral philosophy to medical ethics by saying that medical ethics is an applied discipline whereas sociology is an academic discipline. He says: 'Ironically, then, it is the medical ethicists, trained in philosophy and theology and given to abstraction, who are often worldly, and it is the sociologists of medical ethics who are often curiously otherworldly' (2000: 7). He argues that whilst the conventional distinction exists between the moral philosophical or normative approach and the social science or empirical approach, the distinction has its shortcomings, and he sees it more as a matter of emphasis than of being entirely empirical or normative. In this view Zussman is with Jennings (1986; 1990) when he goes on:

> For the philosophers it is typically enough to know that a phenomenon exists, regardless of the distributions that often obsessively occupy the social scientist. Similarly, social scientists seem capable of only a fairly limited range of normative claims: deontological arguments, based on judgements about the moral character of an act, are almost entirely absent from social scientific thought. (2000: 8)

Zussman (2000) along with others makes the point that the expectation is that social science is needed to help out bioethics in some way. Hoffmaster wrote a paper entitled 'Can ethnography save the life of medical ethics?' (1992), and later in his *Bioethics in social context* (2001) envisaged a larger role for social science. In Zussman's assessment:

> Hoffmaster's argument constitutes a virtual manifesto for a sociology of medical ethics and deserves extended consideration. At the center of his argument is a critique of an 'applied ethics' model. Rather than a style of ethics that begins with a few basic principles and then attempts to apply them across a wide range of circumstances, Hoffmaster is suggesting a style of ethical reasoning that works from the ground up, based in dense local knowledge of particular social situations ... Hoffmaster assigns a special place to ethnography. Indeed, if we were to take Hoffmaster's suggestions seriously, medical ethics would become a very different enterprise. The boundaries between social science and philosophy, between the normative and the empirical, would come close to disappearing. (2000: 10)

Hoffmaster says that as bioethics has been concerned with theoretical justifications, social science has stayed at the margins of the bioethics enterprise. Bioethics is concerned with the normative 'oughts' and social science with descriptive ethics. It is interesting to note that Hoffmaster's call for a consideration of context, whilst different, is not so far removed from Aristotle's idea of the importance of context in the arrival at sound moral judgements. Thompson et al. sum up this position in this way: 'Aristotle and the advocates of a prudential and casuistic approach to ethics are concerned to emphasise that decisions always relate to specific individuals acting in particular situations' (2000: 305).

Sociological analysis of intensive care work allows us to draw some conclusions about the wider effects of intensive care on the work of professionals and hospitals (Anspach 1987; Chambliss 1996; Melia 2001; Zussman 1992). Whilst the ICU is regarded as a distinctive locale by those who work in it, and indeed by the rest of the hospital, intensive care practices provide a more generalisable model for teamwork and consensus practice in other areas, where clinical decisions are difficult and interprofessional differences of opinion exist. The lessons that we can draw from intensive care would suggest that medical ethics and nursing ethics might be better played out as health care ethics. This formulation puts the patient in the centre and emphasises the importance of interdisciplinary teamwork in a system where medicine has the legal responsibility for the clinical diagnosis and treatment decisions in patient care, yet nursing plays a crucial care and organisational role. The separatist configuration of medical ethics and nursing ethics has served to perpetuate the differences between the two groups, rather than to suggest ways of interprofessional co-operation, whilst maintaining the professional integrity of the two occupational groups.

It seems then that there are central features of intensive care practice, both organisational and clinical, which, far from setting it apart from the rest of the hospital, make it an obvious blueprint for practice elsewhere. Multiprofessional teamwork works well in the ICU. Working closely together and having an understanding of one another's roles make a good starting point for the ethical discussions that arise in the course of clinical judgement and decision making. As we have seen in earlier chapters, even when there is disagreement, a team which works together has practised and collegial ways of discussing issues together. The team members may come from different disciplines but they come up against the same problems. It can then, as we have said, reasonably be argued that the skills required for good multidisciplinary teamwork are those which can usefully be brought to ethical debate.

PRACTICAL WISDOM AND CLINICAL JUDGEMENT

The team is concerned with the best outcome for patients. How their care is planned and effected has less to do with the preferences of individual professional groups and more to do with how best the different aspects of care can be brought together. To say that the team is more than the sum of its parts is rather hackneyed, but nonetheless true. However, to state this is only to make half of the case for teamwork and a multidisciplinary approach to health care ethics. Equally important is the habit of working together as a team. This habituation of working physically together in a team effort in intensive care also allows for the development of a team approach to handling the ethical issues.

Aristotle argued that the *habit* of doing good brought about the situation where a person could do their best. Aristotle's approach to ethics takes account of context. Rather than simply applying ethical theories to situations or deducing from the major theoretical positions what the best action would be, each case is considered in the context of the situation. In this way the ethical process and the need for a judgement has much in common with clinical judgement. It is in this connection that practical wisdom is a useful notion. In Aristotle's *Nicomachean ethics* (trans. 1976) he defines what he calls *phronesis* as 'practical wisdom, prudence and common sense'. One of Aristotle's ideas which has utility in terms of health care ethics comes in his writing about habituation. He says that 'moral virtues, like crafts, are acquired by practice and habituation' (Book II, 1103 a14–b1). A virtue in the ancient Greek world was an excellence, not dissimilar from our notion of competence. In an uncannily relevant example of prudence, or practical wisdom, Aristotle says:

> Prudence is not concerned with universals only; it must also take cognizance of particulars, because it is concerned with conduct, and conduct has its sphere in particular circumstances. That is why some people who do not possess [theoretical] knowledge are more effective in action (especially if they are experienced) than others who do possess it. For example, suppose that someone knows that light flesh foods are digestible and wholesome, but does not know what kinds are light; he will be less likely to produce health than one who knows that chicken is wholesome. But prudence is practical, and therefore it must have both kinds of knowledge, or especially the latter. (Book VI 1141 b8–27)

Thompson et al. say that Aristotle's ethics

> combines the emphasis of virtue ethics on the integrity and competence of the moral agent with a detailed analysis of the virtues (or competencies) necessary for sound moral judgement and effective moral action. (2000: 305)

All of this has a surprisingly contemporary ring to it, and is perhaps one explanation for the popularity of the Aristotelian approach to ethical debate in health care. The increasing focus on competencies in both medical and nursing education adds weight to the argument for an interprofessional approach to learning and to ethical debate in the context of health care delivery. Aristotle's thesis is that ethical virtues are instilled in people by habit, they are not in us by nature. Virtues, or states of character, are acquired by undertaking the virtuous acts as one would do if one already had the state of character. A similar approach is taken to becoming a professional, nurse or doctor: there is a lot of what sociologists call 'anticipatory socialisation' (Becker et al. 1961; Melia 1987; Merton et al. 1957). Teamwork brings with it understandings of each member's practice and thinking, so that when it comes to the moral dimension of care there is some basis upon which to proceed. This understanding paves the way for working towards health care ethics, rather than discipline-specific ethics. Health care ethics moves the focus away from the professions and towards a patient-centred health care.

This book is, among other things, about exploring the question of what sociology and moral philosophy have to offer when it comes to ethics in health care. The debates about bioethics and the social sciences tend to range around the idea that they have something to offer each other but there are also reservations about whether an emphasis on context and experience detracts from ethics. Callahan's (1999) remark about ethics having to be ethics, not sociology and not medicine, sums this position up. It is perhaps worth saying, however, that aside from this difficult ground there is a clear place for sociology, and social sciences more generally, in the field of bioethics – and that is to supply the methods and techniques of empirical work. Philosophers may be basing their consequentialist arguments upon assumptions or assertions which have not been empirically tested. If the premise turns out to be false then the whole argument is destabilised. Zussman (2000: 10) notes that if the task of social science amounts to no more than undertaking the empirical work in ethics then it is something of a junior partner. Zussman argues, with Hoffmaster (1992), that social science can do more: it can offer insights into how moral problems are 'perceived and constructed by those whom they affect and how these individuals handle these problems' (2000: 10). The converse is also true, in so far as moral philosophy can make useful commentary on the sociological analysis of health care.

The sociological analysis of intensive care work (Anspach 1987; Chambliss 1996; Melia 2001; Seymour 2000; Zussman 1992) provides insights into how issues which a philosopher would regard as matters of right and wrong are handled in clinical situations. The sociological approach to ethical issues in health care provides a particular kind of empirical approach to understanding intensive care work and the moral dimension of care. The bioethics literature is increasingly concerned with empirical studies in contrast to the theoretical philosophical papers which used to predominate. The empirical work is concerned with topics such as medical errors, patient complaints, informed consent, clinical trials, staffing levels and their implications for care. Along with these studies the literature covers issues which we are accustomed to finding in ethical debate in health care: these include end-of-life decisions, dignity in terminal illness, abortion, patients' rights and so on.[3] The sociological studies allow us to understand how the social practices which surround clinical practice play out. We must understand clinical practice as it is, rather than starting out with the more overtly philosophical positions on how things 'ought' to be. The philosophical approach would tend to apply philosophical theory to clinical decisions, for example taking a utilitarian or deontological approach. The insights yielded through sociological analysis are useful to the health care ethics project. The descriptions of teamwork suggest that there is an understanding by health care professionals of each other's disciplines and views in ethical debates. As we suggested in Chapter 1, the old divisions between the different professional groups, notably nursing and medicine, are less relevant to multiprofessional work practices.

A collaborative approach to health care ethics is essential in a health care system which is trying to put patients first and to respect their rights. Indeed the original model of medical ethics with nursing ethics sitting alongside seemed to propel nursing into the position of some kind of counterweight or corrective to medical practice and ethics. Nursing could be said to have compounded this by adopting the rather doubtful role of patients' advocate. An adversarial relationship between the two professions is not conducive to the empowerment of patients, nor is it, as we have stressed elsewhere, especially collegial. Indeed a combination of the nurse as advocate and the increasing appearance of the patient as litigant threatens to destroy the patient-centred, multidisciplinary health service ideal.

APPLIED ETHICS

The main players in health care – medicine and nursing – are practice disciplines which draw on sciences, but they are not in themselves sciences. Medicine and nursing draw on various social and biomedical sciences. It is interesting to note that when health care professions draw on moral philosophy they do not use the literature, theoretical insights and methods in the same way that the moral philosopher would. Health care professionals have certain professional expectations and commitments to meet and so in terms of moral choices some options are precluded. These are options which a philosopher carrying out a conventional philosophical analysis would be able to suggest, for example, utilitarian-driven euthanasia, or not providing neonatal intensive care. The point is that medicine and nursing are not disciplines but practices which draw on a range of social and biomedical sciences and on moral philosophy. Callahan noted the proliferation of courses on ethics along with debate about their purpose, and asked, 'Is their aim good behavior, a virtuous life, or sharp ethical analysis?' (1999: 275). Medicine and nursing draw on moral philosophy to further their own purposes. In other words, practice disciplines are following their own agendas and these are therefore limited or at least different from those of the disciplines upon which they draw.4 The moral philosopher can take the argument to its logical conclusion and question society's practices in relation to the conclusions drawn. Health care professionals have limits placed upon them, such that even to voice theoretical possibilities might constitute at the very least poor conduct and at worst rock public trust in health care professionals.

There is some kind of link to be made between the relationship of medicine to moral philosophy and the relationship of medicine to medical sociology. When medicine draws upon moral philosophy or sociology, what is it actually doing? How far can practice disciplines make use of academic ones without distorting the latter beyond their proper limits? In Chapter 4, for instance, the sociology of the body literature offered little that was helpful to the health care ethics project. It was more the methods of the discipline of sociology that shed some light on the moral questions which arise in caring for bodies than it was the product of the sociological enterprise, namely a theory of the body. The goals of the academic disciplines are theoretical development, whereas those of the practice disciplines concern guidance for action. Practical wisdom and clinical judgement sit closely together. Callahan remarks that:

> Sociology and anthropology can offer useful methods for under-
> standing culture and the social determinants of values, and they
> might – though this has not been done so far as I know – have
> something to say about the contextual setting of different ethical
> theories that have appeared in recent years. (1999: 285)

In the early days of medical sociology, Straus (1957) made the distinction between the *sociology of medicine* and *sociology in medicine*. Sociology in medicine refers to work which serves medicine's own preoccupations and needs, whilst the sociology of medicine takes a more structural functional approach and regards the organisation, structures and practices of medicine as matters for study. The sociology of medicine is clearly a more critical enterprise, concerning itself with medical dominance, with medicine as an instrument of social control, and with questioning the scope and boundaries of medical practice. Horobin, in addressing the uncertain role of medical sociology, said rather astutely that it lay 'between the citadel of medicine and the suburb of sociology' (1985: 95). He proposed *sociology with medicine* as a preferable alternative to Straus's distinction.

A similar point, but in this case in connection with the relationship of ethics to medicine, was made by the philosopher William May (1980). He described the plight of the ethicist in these memorable terms: 'the applied ethicist carries water from wells he has not dug to fires he cannot find. He does not seem to be a serious intellectual figure' (1980: 239). The argument is that it is as if health care professionals, when they draw on moral philosophy, are somehow not 'doing philosophy properly', or at least they are doing something different from whatever a philosopher would do. The other side of the coin is that moral philosophers have the luxury of taking the argument to the end conclusion because they are not practising health care and so are free of professional demands and constraints. In different ways Horobin and May are commenting on the limits that the disciplines and practices which constitute health care are working within. The philosopher who works at the well, to follow May's analogy, has far greater freedom to go where philosophical analysis leads. Nevertheless the point about the necessarily slightly paler version of moral philosophy which health care professionals apply is well drawn.

Whatever the utility of ethics when it is applied by health care professionals, the argument in its favour is that drawing on the discipline of moral philosophy, limited though it has to be, brings the language of the reasoning and arguments of philosophy to bear on the issues raised in health care. It provides a starting point and a language to proceed in. It helps to clarify some of the positions adopted by health care professionals in order to come to decisions or accept difficult and unavoidable circumstances. The different shades of argument allow colleagues to see that there often are no clear answers, or no answers at all. This in itself is a useful lesson and leads to a view that it can be regarded as progress to learn to live with uncertainty rather than to be permanently undermined by being uncertain. This is particularly relevant in the ICU in connection with the issue of withholding or withdrawal of treatment. Given what we have said about the impact that the existence of intensive care has on health care activity, the lessons concerning uncertainty are equally important in other areas of care, especially in relation to questions for transfer to ICU or not: in other words, in relation to the question of withholding treatment or not.

Gerhardt makes a helpful comment pertinent to this discussion in connection with the argument for sociology being a legitimate and useful discipline for medicine to draw upon:

> sociology is an *analytical* science while medicine is a *practical* endeavour. The latter may avail itself of various insights of the former, if they are carefully researched. But never should sociology which, within the confines of medicine, is at best one of its theoretical disciplines attempt to overcome or replace medicine. The danger in such an undertaking is that sociology itself forgoes its roots and abandons its tenable aims. Its roots are in the theoretical reflection of societal goings-on. Its tenable aims are the systematic description and methodical explanation of social life and social structures. (1989: 351)

Similarly in the case of moral philosophy being drawn upon by health care ethics, there are limits for the practice discipline. The prime purpose is to assist with the moral aspects of clinical decision making and management of care more generally.

There has to be room for professional judgement and the need to put the patient in the centre. Also there is the need to regulate the professions in which society puts its trust. The lesson from intensive care is that in the ideal form of teamwork that is to be found in the ICU there is an automatic working together, and this includes discussion of the ethical dimension of care. Rather than going forward with different tribes – medicine and nursing – each developing their own professional codes of ethics and literature, it makes sense to move together with a multidisciplinary approach to health care ethics.

COLLABORATION, TEAMWORK AND ETHICS

A collaborative approach to health care ethics sits well with current health care working practices and management strategies in the modernised National Health Service in the UK. In the British NHS there are changes afoot which will work in favour of breaking down these traditional barriers and introduce new ways of working with an emphasis upon teamwork and an open approach to patient-led care. One of the important aspects of the modernised health service is the concept of clinical governance by which all those contributing to health care are deemed to be responsible for ensuring the quality of the care. This approach underlines a joint approach to care and encourages flexible working practices which put the patient at the centre of things and tailor the various professional contributions to best suit the patient.

Clinical governance has been defined as 'corporate accountability for clinical performance' (Scottish Office and Department of Health 1997). The Minister for Health of the day said of it:

> Clinical governance will not replace professional self regulation and individual clinical judgement, concepts that lie at the heart of health care in this country. But it will add an extra dimension that will provide the public with guarantees about standards of clinical care.[5]

Whilst this is essentially an organisational system for delivering quality care, it also points the way for a similar approach to the handling of the moral dimension of care and confronting the ethical decisions which arise in practice. This comes back to the point that we have made already: if you can do teamwork you can do ethics.

As we have seen, it is only with a detailed sociological analysis of how intensive care works that we begin to understand the subtleties of interaction between the professional groups which depend upon each other in order to carry out their role in health care. The old argument about the professional dominance of medicine only takes us so far in understanding how it is that the dynamics of the relationship between medicine and nursing work. In a hierarchical sense medicine has the power, yet in a day to day sense and by the nature of the work it is sometimes nursing that seems to call the shots, as it were (Allen 1997; Chambliss 1996; Melia 2001). When it comes to ethical issues we move into difficult territory. In a very general sense there is no hierarchy in the moral positions taken by members of the team. The balance of ethical analysis does not depend upon the technical or scientific expertise possessed by the holder of a particular moral view. All opinions on the team carry equal weight in a moral sense; it is the social processes which promote consensus that are important to the smooth running of the ICU. Knowing how to disagree and continue to function as a team is the key to getting through the difficult moral terrain of health care.

Great importance is placed on consensus in moral decisions taken in the ICU (Melia 2001; Zussman 1992). Chambliss (1996: 96) has argued that nurses sometimes resort to a moral agenda when the issue in question is one of power. Nurses often use the fact of their proximity to the bedside and more sustained contact with the patient and family as a justification for having a more accurate idea of the patient's wishes. This argument is sometimes shored up by the straw man of a distinction made between care and cure, where the caring role is ascribed to nursing whilst the impression is created of a lack of care in the cure-oriented medical staff. Chambliss notes that: 'Care, some nurses say, distinguishes nursing from medicine: "Nurses care, doctors cure"; and while physicians might dispute the moral connotations of that slogan, few would completely deny its message' (1996: 63).

This stance is not, as I argued earlier, helpful and it does not sit well with teamwork. It is not a useful argument to say that nurses have a 'harder ethical time of it' by virtue of their proximity to the patients. This has to be set against the different but equal burden of doctors having several cases on their minds without being present at the bedside the whole time. This is the lot of senior doctors. In each case there is a moral burden, and the difference between them seems to highlight the fact that the two professions depend upon each other's input in order to be able to carry out their own work. Chambliss describes the difference between the nursing and medical view when he talks of

> the physician's sense of legal and personal responsibility for the case, the nurse's round-the-clock witnessing of the patient's suffering and the family's wishes, or the physician's strong orientation to the physiological outcomes rather than the personal experience of the patient. (1996: 101)

Amid the complex doings of the ICU there are mixed ambitions and expectations in nursing. Nurses want interprofessional co-operation, they have a need to be independent, but there is also perhaps a reluctance to take on the responsibility that goes with that independence. Medical dominance (Freidson 1970) is now in many ways an old idea. Such analysis can provide a refuge for nursing, but it can also be a threat to nursing. It can be said to suit nursing's occasional ambivalence about taking responsibility. So simply resorting to the 'it is the power relationships' argument to explain everything does not work. Negotiated order and the interdependence and overlapping of the work of nursing and medicine are nearer the mark. The modernising of the NHS, with its patient focus and openness, rather leaves behind the old analyses that rely very heavily on dominance and hierarchy. Nursing's professionalising project, the need for medicine to be more open and publicly accountable, along with the general complexity of ICU, all lead to a team approach to health care – teams in which there is respect for the role and opinion of each member.

With the increasing recourse to law in clinical judgements, medicine is rather less powerful than it was. Zussman (1992: 151) argues that medicine initially tried to turn technical issues into ethical ones and now can be found turning ethical matters into technical ones. The increasingly educated public and the media attention that is paid to health care matters create a difficult tension between society wanting knowledgeable professional groups that it can trust and, in the case of medicine, identifying a profession as too powerful and not sufficiently open. The inquiries following the organ retention scandal at Alder Hey Hospital (Redfern Report 2001) and the unacceptably high mortality rate in paediatric cardiac surgery at Bristol Royal Infirmary (Kennedy Report 2001) led to a wave of public mistrust in health care and the medical profession in particular and changes in the law (see Chapter 4). In this connection Zussman's (1992) view is interesting. He says that whilst it is medicine's opinion that it is limited by law, in practice this is not so much the case:

> Because physicians resent any interference with their discretion, they exaggerate the limited interference that the law does represent. The irony is that physicians, in their resentment of legal interference, make the law's influence greater than it would otherwise be. (1992: 185)

Zussman is commenting on the American system, but the view would stand also, if to a lesser degree, in the UK. Windeyer may have been right when, in making the point that the law is perhaps more sympathetic to medicine's position than the medical profession thinks to be the case, he commented that we have a situation of 'Law, marching with medicine but in the rear and limping a little'.[b]

Whatever the result of academic disciplines being drawn upon by the practices within health care, it remains the case that there will be differences between what sociologists and moral philosophers will argue and how the health care professionals will use or apply sociology and moral philosophy to their practices. One thing is for sure: once these disciplines have been drawn upon or applied, particularly in the field of professional judgement, they will continue to be used. As Zussman puts it: 'For better or for worse – or for both – medical ethics has entered the discourse of medical practice' (1992: 229).

In the case of health care ethics I would make a similar point for the disciplines of sociology and moral philosophy. Callahan (1999) talks of bioethics being dominated by the 'troika' of medicine, law and philosophy. In twenty-first century health care ethics it is perhaps more of a foursome – health care professionals, the law, sociology and moral philosophy – as the practice disciplines strive to work within the framework of good practice, quality care and the law.

If we look at how this foursome works out in terms of patient needs, we find that the practice is rather more complex than the wiring diagram would suggest. We have the patient with needs and rights, characterised as 'I want such and such a treatment, and I would like it now.' The health care professionals have the service to offer: they make professional clinical judgements which on Zussman's (1992) analysis can in some cases be regarded as 'technical' and free of legal or philosophical interference. Then we have the moral philosophical view on what is right or wrong, good or bad. These judgements are made according to rules, principles and ethical theory. The law brings a different perspective, with legal positions and case law testing new ground. Sociological analysis, which completes the foursome, can show that the context of practice proves to be a rather messier and uncertain business than the moral philosophers or the law courts, and indeed medical science, would have it seem.

The health care professionals trying to follow the guidance of health care ethics have to make the best of the clinical situation in which they find themselves. They move back and forth between the more and less certain pronouncements of medical science, moral philosophy and the law, and arrive at clinical judgement and action which have to meet patient approval, professional standards and legal requirements. The clinical world, well exemplified by the ICU, is one of messy compromise and negotiation and is always unpredictable and uncertain.

Aristotle's approach to working out what is the good thing to do by taking account of the situation and arriving at the best answer in that particular instance – his practical wisdom – is very close to clinical judgement. We may set out with a clear theoretical view of what is the right thing to do, but circumstances may cause us to adjust and negotiate towards a better solution for the case. This brings us back to the point made by Boyd (1999), which is that in the end patients are in the hands of health care professionals and have to rely on their integrity and good moral judgement. Ultimately patients must rely on, in Boyd's words, 'the scientific and humane clinical judgement of the doctors and nurses into whose care the patient is delivered' (1999: 7). For this reason it is essential that we have ongoing debate and analysis – philosophical, legal and sociological – so that health care professionals can reflect on practice and consult a reliable literature when they wish to inform their practice. My argument throughout this book has been that as this practice is increasingly to be undertaken in teams, a joint approach to health care ethics is an obvious route to take.

NOTES

1   Hochschild (1983) talks of 'emotional work' and Strauss et al. (1985) describe 'sentimental work', all referring to what has for a long while been thought of as 'tender loving care' or bedside manner.

2   In the context of a discussion of managed clinical networks, Lapsley and Melia (2001) note that the 'strength of weak ties' should not be underestimated, that is the strength of professional disciplines over the day to day work organisation.

3   See for example the review of empirical studies in bioethics in the *Bulletin of Medical Ethics* January 2003 no. 184 pp. 13–22.

4   I am grateful to Kenneth Boyd for sparking these ideas about the interrelationship between sciences and practice. I am, though, responsible for the views expressed here.

5   Galbraith, Management Executive Letter 'Clinical governance', 1998.

6   The quotation comes from the case *Mount Isa Mines* v. *Pusey* (1970) 125 CLR 383, 395 per Windeyer J. This judgement was made in the High Court of Australia (in the appeal).

references

Adrian, W., Kinirons, M. and Stewart, K. (1995) 'Cardiopulmonary resuscitation: doctors and nurses expect too much', *Journal of the Royal College of Physicians*, 29: 20–4.

Ahmedzai, S. (1996) 'Making sense out of life's failure', *Progress in Palliative Care*, 4: 1–3.

Allen, D. (1997) 'The nursing–medicine boundary: a negotiated order?', *Sociology of Health and Illness*, 19 (4): 498–520.

Anspach, R. (1987) 'Prognostic conflict in life and death decisions: the organization as an ecology of knowledge', *Journal of Health and Social Behaviour*, 28: 215–31.

Aristotle (trans. 1976) 'Nicomachean ethics', in J.A.K. Thomson (trans.), *The ethics of Aristotle, rev. edn*. Harmondsworth: Penguin.

Ashby, M. (1998) 'Palliative care, death causation, public policy and the law', *Progress in Palliative Care*, 6: 69–77.

Atkinson, P. (1984) 'Training for certainty', *Social Science and Medicine*, 19: 949–56.

Atkinson, P. (1995) *Medical Talk and Medical Work: The Liturgy of the Clinic*. London: Sage.

Atkinson, S., Bihari, D., Smithies, M., Daly, K., Mason, R. and McColl, I. (1994) 'Identification of futility in intensive care', *Lancet*, 344: 1203–4.

Audit Commission (1999) *Critical to Success: The Place of Efficient and Effective Critical Care Services Within the Acute Hospital*. London: Audit Commission.

Backett-Milburn, K. and McKie, L. (eds) (2001) *Constructing Gendered Bodies*. Basingstoke: Palgrave.

Baldock, G., (1995) 'Medicine and the media: an everyday story of ICU folk', *British Medical Journal*, 310: 1612–13.

Beauchamp, T.L. and Childress, J.F. (1989) *Principles of Biomedical Ethics, 3rd edn*. Oxford: Oxford University Press.

Beauchamp, T.L. and Childress, J.F. (1994) *Principles of Biomedical Ethics, 4th edn*. Oxford: Oxford University Press.

Beauchamp, T.L. and Childress, J.F. (2001) *Principles of Biomedical Ethics, 5th edn*. Oxford: Oxford University Press.

Becker, H.S., Geer, B., Hughes, E.C. and Strauss, A.L. (1961) *Boys in White*. Chicago: University of Chicago Press.

Bennett, D. and Bion, J. (1999) 'Organisation of intensive care', *British Medical Journal*, 318: 1468–70.

Bion, J. (1995) 'Editorial. Rationing intensive care', *British Medical Journal*, 310: 682–3.

Biswas, B. (1999) 'Medicalization: a nurse's view', in D. Clark and J. Seymour (eds), *Reflections on Palliative Care*. Buckingham: Open University Press.

Bourdieu, P. (1988) *Language and Symbolic Power*. Cambridge: Polity Press.

Boyd, K.M. (1999) 'Advance directives: the ethical implications', *Scottish Journal of Healthcare Chaplaincy*, 2: 3–7.

Boyd, K.M. (2002) 'Editorial. The law, death and medical ethics: Mrs Pretty and Ms B', *Journal of Medical Ethics*, 28 (4): 211–12.

British Medical Association (1993) *Medical Ethics Today: Its Practice and Philosophy*. London: BMJ Publishing Group.

British Medical Association (1994) 'Guidelines on treatment decisions for patients in a persistent vegetative state', *Medical Ethics Committee*. London: BMA.

British Medical Association (1995) *Advance Statements About Medical Treatment: Code of Practice with Explanatory Notes*. London: BMJ Publishing Group.

British Medical Association (1999, update 2001) *Withholding and Withdrawing Life-prolonging Medical Treatment: Guidance for Decision Making*. London: BMJ Books.

Brody, H. (1994) 'The four principles and narrative ethics', in R. Gillon and A. Lloyd (eds), *Principles of Health Care Ethics*. Chichester: Wiley.

Brody, H. (1997) 'Medical futility: a useful concept', in M.B. Zucker and H.D. Zucker (eds), *Medical Futility and the Evaluation of Life-sustaining Interventions*. Cambridge: Cambridge University Press.

Bucher, R. and Strauss, A.L. (1961) 'Professions in process', *American Journal of Sociology*, 66: 325–34.

Bulletin of Medical Ethics (2000) 'News: competant patients decide their treatment', *Bulletin of Medical Ethics*, 176: 5–6.

Callahan, D. (1999) 'The social sciences and the task of bioethics', *Daedalus*, 128 (4): 275–94.

Campbell, A.V. (1984) *Moral Dilemmas in Medicine*. Edinburgh: Churchill Livingstone.

Campbell, A.V., Charlesworth, M., Gillett, G. and Jones, G. (1997) *Medical Ethics*. Oxford: Oxford University Press.

Capron, A.M. (1997) 'Foreword', in M.B. Zucker and H.D. Zucker (eds), *Medical Futility and the Evaluation of Life-sustaining Interventions*. Cambridge: Cambridge University Press.

Chambliss, D. (1996) *Beyond Caring: Hospitals, Nurses and the Social Organisation of Ethics*. Chicago: University of Chicago Press.

Clark, D. and Seymour, J. (1999) *Reflections on Palliative Care*. Buckingham: Open University Press.

Comte, A. (ed. 1975) *The essential writings*, ed. G. Lenzer. New York: Harper and Row.

Conference of Medical Royal Colleges and their Faculties in the UK (1976) 'Diagnosis of brain death', *British Medical Journal*, 2 November: 1187–8.

Conference of Medical Royal Colleges and their Faculties in the UK (1979) 'Diagnosis of death', *British Medical Journal*, 1 February: 332.

Daly, K., Beale, R. and Chang, R.W.S. (2001) 'Reduction in mortality after inappropriate early discharge from intensive care unit: logistic regression triage model', *British Medical Journal*, 322: 1274.

Department of Health (1996) *Guidelines on Admission to and Discharge from Intensive Care and High Dependency Units*. London: Department of Health.

Department of Health (1997) *The New NHS: Modern, Dependable.* Cm 3807. London: The Stationery Office.

Department of Health (1998) *The New NHS: Working Together. Securing a Quality Workforce for the NHS.* London: Department of Health.

Department of Health (1999) 'Review of Nurses, Midwives and Health Visitors Act: government response to the recommendations', *Health Service Circular,* 1999/030. London: Department of Health.

Department of Health (2000) *The NHS Plan: a Plan for Investment, a Plan for Reform.* London: The Stationery Office.

DHSS (1979) *The Removal of Cadaveric Organs for Transplantation: A Code of Practice.* London: HMSO.

Descartes, R. (trans. 1988) *Descartes: Selected Philosophical Writings,* trans. and ed. J. Cottingham, R. Stoothoff and D. Murdoch. Cambridge: Cambridge University Press.

Downie, R.S. (1996) 'Introduction to medical ethics', in N. Pace and S. McLean (eds), *Ethics and the Law in Intensive Care.* Oxford: Oxford University Press.

Doyle, D., Hanks, G.W.C. and MacDonald, N. (1993) *Oxford Textbook of Palliative Care.* Oxford: Oxford University Press.

Durkheim, E. (1952) *Suicide: a study in sociology* (1897). London: Routledge and Kegan Paul.

Engelhardt, H.T. (1988) 'Re-examining the definition of death and becoming clearer about what it is to be alive', in R.M. Zander (ed.), *Death: Beyond Whole Brain Criteria.* Dordrecht: Reidel.

Etzioni, A. (1975) *A Comparative Analysis of Complex Organisations* (1961). New York: Free Press.

Feher, M. (1989) *Fragments for a History of the Body, parts I–III.* New York: Zone.

Fox, R. (1957) 'Training for uncertainty', in R.K. Merton, G. Reader and P.L. Kendall (eds), *The Student Physician.* Cambridge, MA: Harvard University Press.

Fox, R. (1959) *Experiment Perilous: Physicians and Patients Facing the Unknown.* Glencoe, IL: Free Press.

Fox, R. (1980) 'The evolution of medical uncertainty', *Milbank Memorial Fund Quarterly,* 58: 1–49.

Fox, R. (1989) *The Sociology of Medicine.* Englewood Cliffs, NJ: Prentice Hall.

Fox, R. and Swazey, J. (1974) *The Courage to Fail, 2nd rev. edn.* Chicago: University of Chicago Press.

Frank, A. (1991) 'For a sociology of the body: an analytic review', in M. Featherstone, M. Hepworth and B.S. Turner (eds), *The Body: Social Processes and Cultural Theory.* London: Sage.

Frankena, W.K. (1973) *Ethics, 2nd edn.* Englewood Cliffs, NJ: Prentice Hall.

Freidson, E. (1970) *Profession of Medicine: A Study of the Sociology of Applied Knowledge.* New York: Dodd, Mead.

Freidson, E. (1994) *Professionalism Reborn: Theory, Prophecy and Policy.* Cambridge: Polity.

Gamarnikow, E. (1991) 'Nurse or woman: gender and professionalism in reformed nursing', in P. Holden and J. Littleworth (eds), *Anthropology and Nursing.* London: Routledge.

Gerhardt, U. (1989) *Ideas About Illness: An Intellectual and Political History of Medical Sociology.* Basingstoke: Macmillan.

Giddens, A. (1977) *Studies in Social and Political Theory.* London: Hutchinson.

Giddens, A. (1979) *Central Problems in Social Theory: Action Structure and Contradiction in Social Analysis.* London: Macmillan.

Giddens, A. (1984) *The Constitution of Society*. Cambridge: Polity.

Giddens, A. (1991) *Modernity and Self-identity: Self and Society in the Late Modern Age*. Cambridge: Polity.

Gillett, G. (1986) 'Why let people die?', *Journal of Medical Ethics*, 12: 83–6.

Gilligan, C. (1977) Concepts of the self and of morality. *Harvard Educational Review*, 47: 481–517.

Gilligan, C. (1982) *In a Different Voice*. Cambridge, MA: Harvard University Press.

Gilligan, C. (1993) 'Reply to critics', in M.J. Larrabee (ed.), *An Ethic of Care: Feminist and Interdisciplinary Perspectives*. London: Routledge.

Gillon, R. (1994) 'The four principles revisited: a reappraisal', in R. Gillon and A. Lloyd (eds), *Principles of Health Care Ethics*. Chichester: Wiley.

Gillon, R. and Lloyd, A. (eds) (1994) *Principles of Health Care Ethics*. Chichester: Wiley.

Glaser, B.G. and Strauss, A.L. (1965) *Awareness of Dying*. Chicago: Aldine.

Glaser, B.G. and Strauss, A.L. (1967) *Discovery of Grounded Theory*. New York: Aldine.

Goffman, E. (1969) *Presentation of Self in Everyday Life*. Harmondsworth: Penguin.

Harvard Medical School (1968) 'A definition of irreversible coma', *Journal of the American Medical Association*, 205 (6): 85–8.

Henderson, V. (1960) *Basic Principles of Nursing Care*. London: ICN.

Henderson, V. (1964) 'The nature of nursing', *American Journal of Nursing*, August: 62–8.

Higginson, I. (1993) 'Palliative care: a review of past changes and future trends', *Journal of Public Health Medicine*, 15: 3–8.

Hoffmaster, B. (1992) 'Can ethnography save the life of medical ethics?', *Social Science and Medicine*, 35: 1421–31.

Hoffmaster, B. (ed.) (2001) *Bioethics in Social Context*. Philadelphia: Temple University Press.

Horobin, G. (1985) 'Medical sociology in Britain: true confessions of an empiricist', *Sociology of Health and Illness*, 7 (1): 94–107.

House of Lords (1994) *Report of the Select Committee on Medical Ethics,Vol. I: Report; Vol II: Oral evidence*. HL Paper 21.1. London: HMSO.

Hughes, E.C. (1951) 'Studying the nurse's work', in E.C. Hughes (ed.), (1971) *The Sociological Eye: Selected Papers*. London: Transaction.

Hughes, E.C. (1958) *Men and Their Work*. Glencoe, IL: Free Press.

Hume, D. (1711–76) *On Human Nature and the Understanding*. Edited by A. Flew (1962). London: Collier McMillan.

Intensive Care Society (1997) *Standards for Intensive Care*. London: Intensive Care Society.

Jennett, B. and Plum, F. (1972) 'Persistent vegetative state after brain damage: a syndrome in search of a name', *Lancet*, 1: 734–7.

Jennett, B. (1984) 'Inappropriate use of intensive care', *British Medical Journal*, 289: 1709–10.

Jennett, B. (1994) 'Medical technology, social and health care issues', in R. Gillon and A. Lloyd (eds), *Principles of Health Care Ethics*. Chichester: Wiley.

Jennett, B. (1996) 'Brain death and the persistent vegetative state', in N. Pace and S. McLean (eds), *Ethics and the Law in Intensive Care*. Oxford: Oxford University Press.

Jennings, B. (1986) 'Applied ethics and the vocation of social science', in J.P. De Marco and R.M. Fox (eds), *New Directions in Ethics: The Challenge of Applied Ethics*. New York: Routledge and Kegan Paul.

Jennings, B. (1990) 'Ethics and ethnography in neo-natal intensive care', in G. Weisz (ed.), *Social Science Perspectives on Medical Ethics*. Dordrecht: Kluwer.

JM Consulting (1996) *The Regulation of Health Professions: Report of a Review of the Professions Supplementary to Medicine Act 1960 with Recommendations for New Legislation*. Bristol: JM Consulting.

JM Consulting (1998) *The Regulation of Nurses, Midwives and Health Visitors: Report on a Review of the Nurses, Midwives and Health Visitors Act 1997*. Bristol : JM Consulting.

Jones, D.G. (2000) *Speaking for the Dead: Cadavers in Biology and Medicine*. Aldershot: Ashgate.

Jonsen, A. (1995) 'Casuistry: an alternative or complement to principles', *Journal of the Kennedy Institute of Ethics*, 5.

Jonsen, A. and Toulmin, S. (1988) *The Abuse of Casuistry: A History of Moral Reasoning*. Berkeley, CA: University of California Press.

Kant, I. (1788) *Foundations of metaphysics of morals*, trans. Lewis White Beck (1959). Indianapolis: Bobbs-Merrill.

Kennedy Report (2001) *Learning from Bristol: the Report of the Public Inquiry into Children's Heart Surgery at the Bristol Royal Infirmary 1984–1995*. Chairman I. Kennedy. Cm 5207. London: Stationery Office.

Kohlberg, L. (1976) 'Moral stages and moralization', in T. Lickona (ed.), *Moral Development and Behavior*. New York: Rinehart and Winston.

Lamb, D. (1996) *Death, Brain Death and Ethics* (1987). Aldershot: Avebury.

Lapsley, I. and Melia, K.M. (2001) 'Clinical actions and financial constraints: the limits to rationing intensive care', *Journal of Sociology of Health and Illness*, 23 (5): 729–46.

Lawler, J. (1991) *Behind the Screens: Nursing, Somology and the Problem of the Body*. Edinburgh: Churchill Livingstone.

Le Fanu, J. (1999) *The Rise and Fall of Modern Medicine*. London: Little, Brown.

Liddle, J., Gilleard, C. and Neil, A. (1994) 'The views of elderly patients and their relatives on cardiopulmonary resuscitation', *Journal of the Royal College of Physicians*, 28: 228–9.

McHaffie, H.E. and Fowlie, P.W. (1996) *Life, Death and Decisions: Doctors and Nurses Reflect on Neonatal Practice*. Cheshire: Hochland and Hochland.

McIntosh, J. (1977) *Communication in a Cancer Ward*. London: Croom Helm.

MacIntyre, A. (1981) *After Virtue*. Notre Dame, IN: Notre Dame University Press.

Mackay, L. (1993) *Conflicts in Care: Medicine and Nursing*. London: Chapman and Hall.

McPherson, K. (2001) 'Safer discharge from intensive care to hospital wards', *British Medical Journal*, 322: 1261–2.

McWhirter, J.P. and Pennington, C.R. (1994) 'Incidence and recognition of malnutrition in hospitals', *British Medical Journal*, 308: 945–8.

Mason, J.K. (1988) *Human Life and Medical Practice*. Edinburgh: Edinburgh University Press.

Mason, J.K. and McCall Smith, R.A. (1999) *Law and Medical Ethics, 5th edn*. Edinburgh: Butterworths.

Mason, J.K., McCall Smith, R.A. and Laurie, G.T. (2002) *Law and Medical Ethics, 6th edn*. Edinburgh: Butterworths.

Mauksch, H. (1966) 'The organisational context of nursing practice', in F. Davis (ed.), *The Nursing Profession: Five Sociological Essays*. London: Wiley.

May, W. (1980) 'Professional ethics: setting, terrain and teacher', in D. Callahan and S. Bok (eds), *Ethics Teaching in Higher Education*. New York:

Plenum.

Mead, G.H. (1934) *Mind, Self and Society*. Chicago, IL: University of Chicago Press.

Melia, K.M. (1987) *Learning and Working: The Occupational Socialization of Nurses*. London: Tavistock.

Melia, K.M. (1989) *Everyday Nursing Ethics*. Basingstoke: Macmillan.

Melia, K.M. (1994) 'The task of nursing ethics', *Journal of Medical Ethics*, 20 (4): 7–11.

Melia, K.M. (2000a) *Data from a Study of Ethical Issues in Intensive Care*. University of Edinburgh.

Melia, K.M. (2000b) 'Intensive care: where nurses count', Managing Budgets in the Intensive Care Unit. *Institute of Public Sector Accounting Research Policy Paper 7*. Edinburgh: University of Edinburgh.

Melia, K.M. (2001) 'Ethical issues and the importance of consensus for the intensive care team', *Social Science and Medicine*, 53: 707–19.

Menzies, I (1970) *A Case Study in the Function of Social Systems as a Defence Against Anxiety*. London: Tavistock.

Merrison Report (1975) *Report of the Committee of Inquiry into the Regulation of the Medical Profession*. Cmnd 6018. London: HMSO.

Merton, R.K., Reader, K. and Kendall, P.L. (1957) *The student physician* (R.K. Merton 1955). Cambridge, MA: Harvard University Press.

Mill, J.S. (1861) 'Utilitarianism', in M. Warnock (ed.), (1962) *Utilitarianism on Liberty: Essay on Bentham*. London: Fontana.

Mollaret, P. and Goulon, M. (1959) 'Le coma depassé', *Revue Neurologique*, 101: 3–15.

Muller, J.H. and Koenig, B. (1988) 'On the boundary of life and death: the definition of dying by medical residents', in M. Lock and D. Gordon (eds), *Biomedicine Examined*. Dordrecht: Kluwer.

NCHSPCS (1995) *Specialist Palliative Care: A Statement of Definitions*. London: National Council for Hospice and Specialist Palliative Care Services.

Nightingale, Florence (1859) *Notes on Nursing: What it is and What it is Not*. London: Harrison.

Nudeshima, J. (1991) 'Obstacles to brain death and organ transplantation in Japan', *Lancet*, 338: 1063.

Pace, N. and McLean, S. (eds) (1996) *Ethics and the Law in Intensive Care*. Oxford: Oxford University Press.

Parsons, T. (1951) *The Social System*. Glencoe, IL: Free Press.

Porter, R. (1997) *The Greatest Benefit to Mankind: A Medical History of Humanity from Antiquity to the Present*. London: Harper Collins.

President's Commission (1982) *Making Health Care Decisions, Vol 1: Report*. President's Commission for the Study of Ethical Problems in Medicine and Biomedical and Behavioral Research. Washington, DC: Government Printing Office.

Ramsey, P. (1978) *Ethics at the Edges of Life: Medical and Legal Intersections*. London: Yale University Press.

Randall, F. and Downie, R.S. (1996) *Palliative Care Ethics: A Good Companion*. Oxford: Oxford University Press

Rawls, J. (1972) *A Theory of Justice*. Oxford: Oxford University Press.

Redfern Report (2001) *Report of the Royal Liverpool Children's Inquiry*. Chair Michael Redfern QC. HC 12–II. London: Stationery Office.

Rosenthal, M. (1995) *The Incompetent Doctor: Behind Closed Doors*. Buckingham: Open University Press.

Roth, J. (1963) *Timetables*. New York: Bobbs-Merrill.

Sage, W.M., Rosenthal, M.H. and Silverman, J.F. (1986) 'Is intensive care worth it? An assessment of input and outcome for the critically ill', *Critical Care Medicine*, 14: 777–82.

Scottish Office and Department of Health (1997) *Designed to Care: Renewing the National Health Service in Scotland*. White Paper. London: The Stationery Office.

Seymour, J.E. (2000) *Critical Moments: Death and Dying in Intensive Care*. Buckingham: Open University Press.

Shilling, C. (1993) *The Body and Social Theory*. London: Sage.

Singer, P. (1994) *Re-thinking Life and Death: The Collapse of Our Traditional Ethics*. Oxford: Oxford University Press.

Singer, P. (2002) 'Ms B and Diane Pretty: a commentary', *Journal of Medical Ethics*, 28 (4): 234–5.

Skegg, P.D.G. (1988) *Law, Ethics and Medicine: Studies in Medical Law*. Oxford: Oxford University Press.

Smith, G. and Neilsen, M. (1999) 'ABC of intensive care: criteria for admission', *British Medical Journal*, 318: 1544–7.

Stacey, M. (1988) *The Sociology of Health and Healing*. London: Unwin Hyman.

Stein, L.I. (1967) 'The doctor–nurse game', *Archives of General Psychiatry*, 16: 699–703.

Stein, L.I., Watts, D. and Howell, T. (1990) 'The doctor–nurse game revisited', *New England Journal of Medicine*, 322 (8): 546–9.

Straus, R. (1957) 'The nature and status of medical sociology', *American Sociological Review*, 22: 200–4.

Strauss, A.L., Schatzman, L., Ehrlich, D., Bucher, R. and Sabshin, M. (1963) 'The hospital and its negotiated order', in E. Freidson (ed.), *The Hospital in Modern Society*. New York: Free Press.

Strauss, A.L. (1978) *Negotiations*. San Francisco: Jossey Bass.

Strauss, A.L., Fagerhaugh, S., Suczec, B. and Wiener, C. (1985) *The Social Organisation of Medical Work*. London: University of Chicago Press.

Task Force (1994) 'The Multi-Society Task Force on Persistent Vegetative State', *New England Journal of Medicine*, 330 (21): 1499–1508.

Thompson, I.E., Melia, K.M. and Boyd, K.M. (2000) *Nursing Ethics, 4th edn*. Edinburgh: Churchill Livingstone.

The Times (1998) 'Ice man', *The Times*, 30 March.

Times Law Report (1998) 'Artist jailed for removing body parts from the anatomy museum of the Royal College of Surgeons in London'.

Toulmin, S. (1981) 'The tyranny of principles', *Hastings Center Report*, 11: 31–9.

Turner, B.S. (1984) *The Body and Society: Explorations in Social Theory*. Oxford: Basil Blackwell.

Turner, B.S. (1987) *Medical Power and Social Knowledge*. London: Sage.

Turner, B.S. (1991) in M. Featherstone, M. Hepworth and B.S. Turner (eds), *The Body: Social Processes and Cultural Theory*. London: Sage.

Turner, B.S. (1992) *Regulating Bodies: Essays in Medical Sociology*. London: Routledge.

Turner, B.S. (1995) *Medical Power and Social Knowledge, 2nd edn*. London: Sage.

Vella, K., Goldfrad, C., Rowan, K., Bion, J. and Black, N. (2000) 'Use of Census development to establish national research priorities in critical care', *British Medical Journal*, 320: 976–78.

Vicinus, M. and Nergaard, B. (eds) (1989) *Ever Yours, Florence Nightingale*. London: Virago.

Walby, S. and Greenwell, J. with Mackay, L. and Soothill, K. (1994) *Medicine and Nursing: Professions in a Changing Health Service*. London: Sage.

Weber, M. (1922) *Economy and Society: An Outline of Interpretive Sociology*, ed. G. Roth and C. Wittich, trans. E. Fischoff (1968). New York: Bedminster.

World Health Organisation (1990) *Cancer Pain Relief and Palliative Care.* Expert Committee. Technical Report Series no. 804. Geneva: WHO.

Wicks, D. (1998) *Nurses and Doctors at Work: Re-thinking Professional boundaries*. Buckingham: Open University Press.

Wikler, D. (1988) 'Not dead, not dying? Ethical categories and persistent vegetative state', *Hastings Center Report*, 18: 41–7.

Winter, B. and Cohen, S. (1999) 'ABC of intensive care: withdrawal of treatment,' *British Medical Journal*, 319: 306–8.

Witz, A. (1992) *Professions and Patriarchy*. London: Routledge.

Zussman, R. (1992) *Intensive Care: Medical Ethics and the Medical Profession.* Chicago: University of Chicago Press.

Zussman, R. (2000) 'The contribution of sociology to medical ethics', *Hastings Center Report*, 30 (1): 7–11.

index

Compiled by INDEXING SPECIALISTS
202 Church Road, Hove, East Sussex BN3 2DJ. Tel: 01273 738299
Website: www.indexing.co.uk